SOMETHING TO STARE AT

JOSH BLUE

SOMETHING TO STARE AT

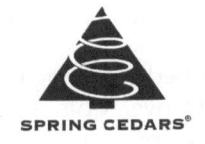

SPRING CEDARS®

This work depicts actual events in the life of the author as truthfully as recollection permits. Some names and identifying characteristics have been changed to protect the privacy of individuals.

Copyright © 2025 by Josh Blue

All rights reserved

First edition, 2025

Cover and book design by Spring Cedars

ISBN 978-1-963117-53-0 (paperback)
ISBN 978-1-963117-54-7 (hardback)
ISBN 978-1-963117-55-4 (ebook)

Published by Spring Cedars
Denver, Colorado
www.springcedars.com

*This book is dedicated to what brings us all together: laughter.
This book is dedicated to the laugh.*

CONTENTS

FOREWORD 1

THE PALSY PUNCH 3

A ROUGH START 7

HIGH SCHOOL 25

EVERGREEN 85

BACK TO AFRICA 103

THE BOOBOO MONKEY 121

THOR IN THE WOODS 143

OFF TO COLORADO 159

COMEDY ACT I 177

SOCCER 203

COMEDY ACT II 241

LAST COMIC STANDING: TRY, TRY AGAIN 257

FINALS 273

THE AFTERMATH 285

ABOUT THE AUTHOR 291

FOREWORD

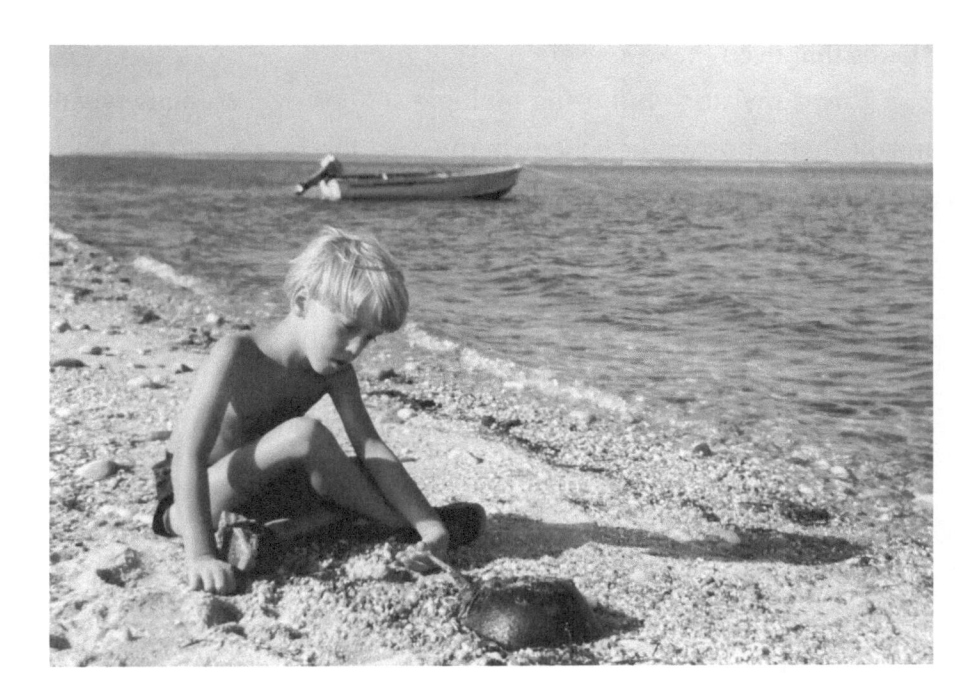

Hello, gentle reader, welcome to my book. If you're not familiar with me, and you perhaps picked this up in an estate sale, I'm Josh Blue—best known for putting the cerebral in cerebral palsy through my stand-up comedy. I'm not writing this foreword to spoil the adventures to come, but to let you in on the laborious process it took to get these words in front of you. Like so many things in my life, I didn't do it alone. I couldn't do it alone. It takes a village to raise an idiot.

It took twenty years to write this book of 300 pages. That averages out to about 15 pages per year! Due to my disability, I'm not able to write or type. I mean, I understand the concept. It just doesn't come out in legible words. I had to employ a small army of scribes to write while I dictated the book, so I've already lost quite a bit of money on this endeavor. My scribe and I would hop on the phone and take it sentence by sentence, with me dictating, and them typing and reading it back, ending with me asking, "Does that even make sense?"

This is my story, but using multiple scribes over so many years meant their ghostwriter echoes permeated the writing. At the end, we had to go back and do it all again to make sure my own voice was the dominant one. I'm also a slow reader, which added time to the painstaking grind of editing. But as you're about to find out, I've overcome far greater obstacles than finishing this book.

And remember: if you don't like something in this book, I blame the scribes—after all, they outnumbered me!

THE PALSY PUNCH

I was apprehensive. It was my first day at junior high school. Up until that point, my peers were disabled kids, and we rode the short bus. Now I was moving on to a school that picked me up in a regular-sized bus, the kind "normal" kids used. My mother drove me to the bus stop in our butternut-squash and brown Volkswagen van, and I asked her to park half a block away. I wanted her in sight, but that didn't mean I was unaware that moms weren't cool.

I stood there with my black backpack and my Mr. T lunch box, which I knew was not cool either. One girl was already there, but she was doing her own thing. I looked in the direction I expected the bus to come from and saw a figure awkwardly working his way toward us. One arm was crooked to his side and twisted up like a chicken wing, and he had a big, wonky limp. I felt relieved; I wouldn't be the only kid in school with cerebral palsy; I wouldn't even be the only disabled kid on the bus.

The boy laboriously crossed the street and walked straight toward me. I called out, "Hey, h-how's it going?"

He laughed and shook his chicken wing of an arm into a regular arm. He straightened his posture and took the slack out of his knee. As he turned his back to me and focused on stomping ants, I chuckled and wondered if he could teach me how to do that until the truth seeped in. By the time I fully realized the boy was just being a cruel dick, the bus had come, and he was already on board. I was glad my mother wasn't close enough to see what had happened; she would have come undone. Part of me wanted to run to the comfort of our ugly van, but I knew I had to face this new reality sooner or later.

The next few months were absolute hell. That bully made fun of me daily, not only on every bus ride, but in the halls as well. He would even follow me home, though we both knew it was out of his way. Then the torture intensified when he discovered the palsied person's kryptonite: The Startle Reflex.

If you scare me, I'll launch through the roof, and it's even worse if I know it's coming. It's as though my body is one giant mousetrap. I'm only telling you this, gentle reader, with the understanding that you will never abuse this knowledge. There's no reason to scare someone with palsy on purpose; you can get enough of a thrill just doing it by accident.

This bully took constant advantage of my hair-trigger mechanics. He would lie in wait and burst out like a jerk-in-the-box, screaming and laughing maniacally as my whole body contorted. He would throw fake punches at me, and my muscles would tense up, painfully. He would slam his heavy biology textbook on the seat behind me, forcing me to seize up and catch air. And perhaps most insidiously, he would sit as close as possible just to fuck with me further. I imagine to outsiders it looked like we were good friends.

One afternoon bus ride, he was sitting across the aisle from me, perched on the edge of his seat. He kept swooping in and yelling, "*Boo!*" I would reliably jump, and he would laugh his evil little laugh. The last time he did it, the mousetrap snapped back. I had a full-body spasm that formed into a directional, well-placed punch to his mouth. It went a bit like this:

"*Boo!*"

Thwack.

He straightened, turned to face forward, and sat for the first time like you're supposed to sit on a bus. He scooted to the window and attended to the business of licking the blood off his teeth. I never heard that evil little laugh directed at me again.

Thus, the Palsy Punch was born. A truly unpredictable force. The marvelous thing about the Palsy Punch is that you don't know where it's coming from.

And neither do I.

A ROUGH START

I was born November 27, 1978, in Cameroon, Central Africa. My dad, Dr. Walter Blue, taught English at a Lutheran mission school in the city of Ngaoundéré. My arrival in Africa was brief, due to a rough C-section after I overstayed my welcome in utero for one month. Because the hospital lacked the proper equipment to induce labor, they performed an emergency eviction. Still the cheapest rent I ever had.

The labor became more dire when the placenta tried to come out first and my mom Jacqui was hemorrhaging. The doctor later said if they had waited thirty minutes longer, I wouldn't have made it, and they probably would have lost my mom, too.

I was not in the clear; I was on oxygen and needed an IV, but the hospital didn't have needles small enough for my baby veins. My outlook was so grim, they baptized me right then and there. Two days after I was born, I showed improvement, and they took me off oxygen. I promptly began to have *grand mal* seizures. In case you don't speak French, gentle reader, those are big, bad seizures.

My mother felt abandoned because her doctor was nowhere to be found. It turned out he ran home to consult his medical books on my mysterious seizures. He later returned to the hospital and gave me a shot of vitamin B12.

I desperately needed more care than this remote, little hospital could offer. My parents devised a plan to get me to America. Nigel, the man who ran the hospital, knew a guy with a bush plane who had once offered its use as a favor. It was time to call in that favor. A group of panicked family friends ventured into the bush to find this man and his plane.

Meanwhile, a nurse named Myrtle Noss brought me to my mother to say goodbye. My condition was so fragile that this was possibly a permanent goodbye. Nurse Noss couldn't bring herself to take me away from my mom; she made my godmother do it.

Early the next morning I was on that bush plane in a wicker basket, accompanied by Nigel, my dad, and nurse Noss. We headed north to Garoua, where we caught a commercial flight south to Yaoundé, the capital. From Yaoundé, we flew to Douala, then on to Paris. From Paris we flew direct to Buffalo, which seems like a weird flight, but maybe it made sense in the '70s.

When we landed in America, we were met by a TV news crew; the story of this troubled baby medevaced out of Africa had beaten me back to the States. I was taken to a hospital for proper care, and when they tested my blood, they discovered I was dangerously low on B12. That shot from the doctor in Africa probably saved my life.

My dad took me out of the hospital to get passport pictures. He explained the situation to the woman taking the photos, and she asked how I had gotten into the States. My dad had carried me in the wicker basket, and I kept quiet through customs. She questioned why no one in New York or Paris had thought to ask about the contents of this wicker basket, adding, "New York is in serious trouble and heads will roll at Charles de Gaulle."

Throughout this entire terrifying adventure, my poor mom was back in Africa, recovering from her brutal C-section, wondering if I was dead or alive. Twelve days after I had been taken in a panic away from her, she returned from lunch with my siblings to find a note in my dad's handwriting tacked on the front door: *Go to nice nurse Noss's house now*.

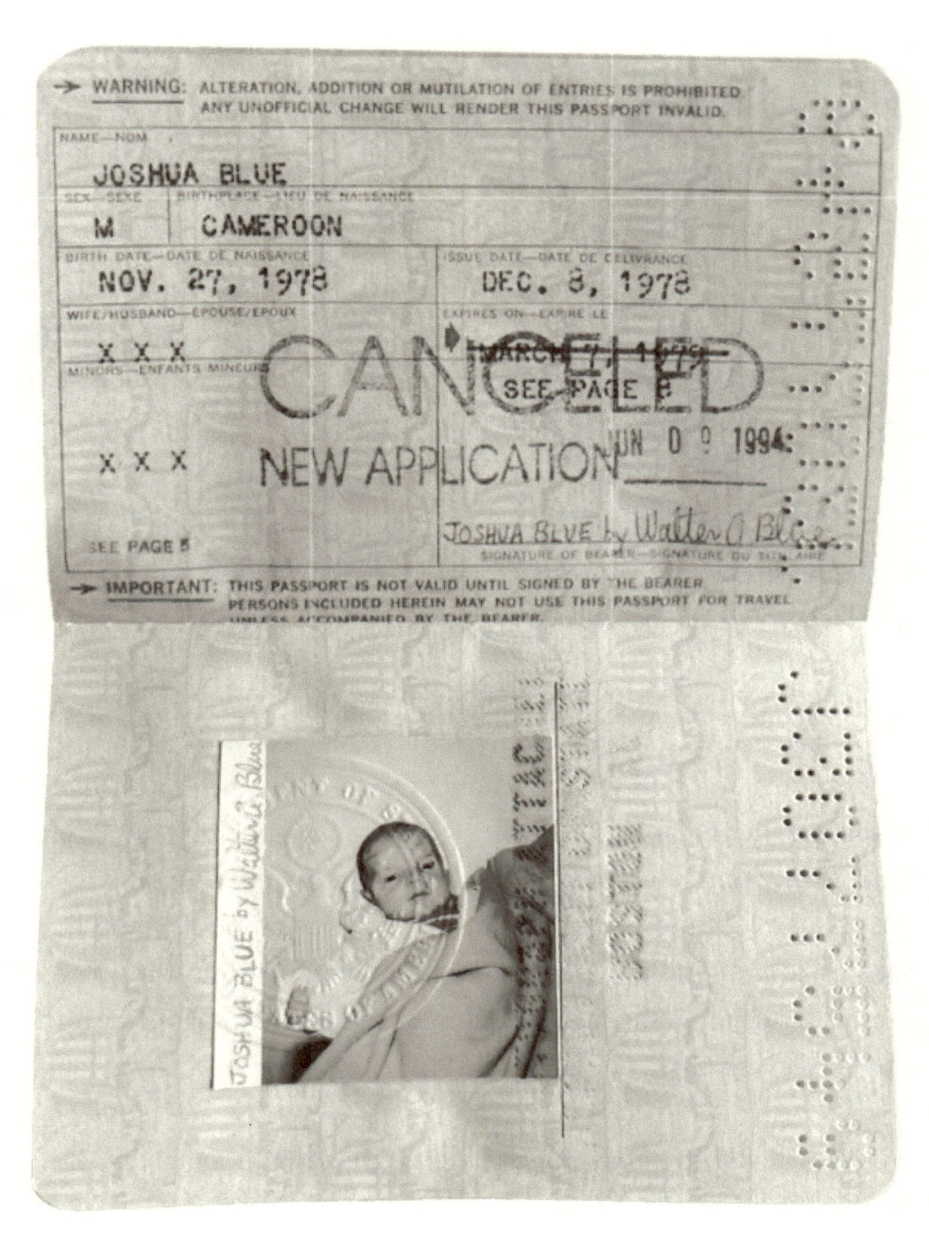

My first mugshot.

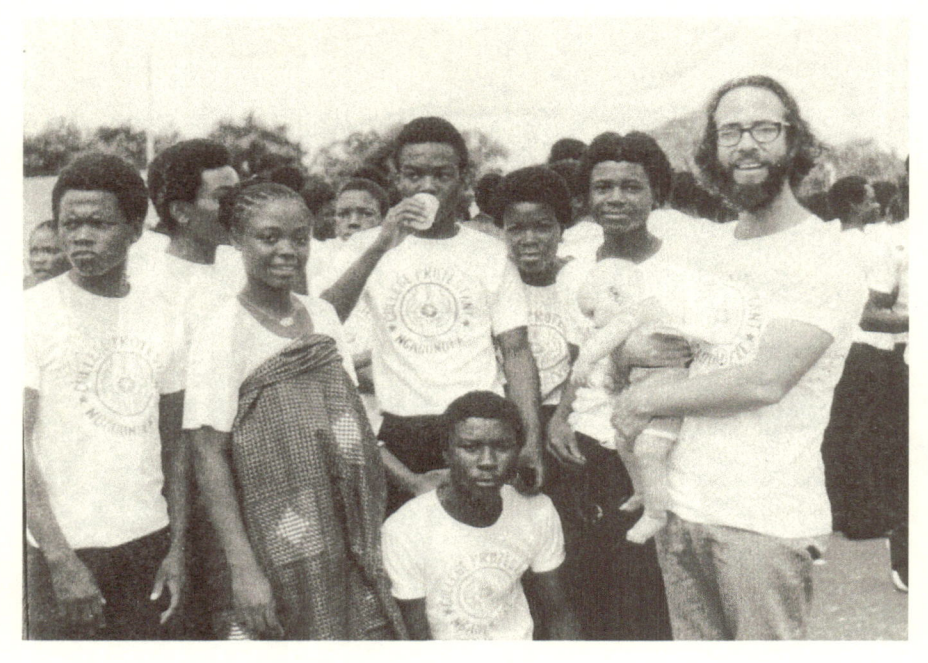

This picture proves I have Black friends.

There I was, stable and back in Africa.

Shortly after I returned, my family traveled with a group of Norwegians through the bush and came upon a village selling exquisite, hand-carved, wooden stools, all made from the same tree. As my dad attempted to negotiate the price, the women and girls began to emerge from their homes. I was an oddity, and they wanted to hold me and pass me around. Despite almost losing me during birth, my mom was not clingy; she let them—to the shock of the Norwegians.

We stayed in Africa for another eight months until my dad's two-year commitment was up, and then my family went back to Saint Paul and resumed their other lives. Technically, they call where we lived The Midway, because it's midway between Minneapolis and St. Paul. It is right on the edge of Frogtown, where the majority of Vietnamese and Hmong refugees settled after the Vietnam war.

We were middle-class, in a not so middle-class house. We were a traditional sit-around-the-dinner-table kind of family, except the chairs at the table were those wooden stools from Cameroon, and we were surrounded by African art and instruments. Visitors observed that our house was like a museum of African artifacts.

My father resumed teaching French and Italian at Hamline University, a few blocks from our house. He is a genius. He speaks thirteen languages, but despite all those languages, I still don't think he can effectively communicate with my mom. His prized possession is a baby grand piano. He would often play classical music or hymns, but his favorite were show tunes. The piano was in the same room as the only TV, and I'd be watching *Garfield*, fighting to hear my show over "A Real Nice Clambake." My dad mainly wore authentic African garb. He was quite the spectacle—a six-foot tall White man with a graying, black beard, wearing a vibrant *dashiki* or *mumu*.

My mom was a stay-at-home mother who ran a home daycare with a small catering business on the side. Later she moved on to being a librarian at my siblings' school. Throughout my childhood, my mother made all my clothes. While other kids were wearing MC Hammer pants, I was sporting homemade Zubaz: atrocious, oversized, stretchy, animal print pants. I remember once she crafted me some pants with street signs saying DON'T DO DRUGS, because I was in a D.A.R.E. class. Sorry Mom, those pants didn't work, but I do wish I had them now! My mother also loved show tunes and always had a snippet of one ready to sing to me for every occasion.

I'm the youngest of four, and I'm glad I was the last child; if I was the first, perhaps my parents would have been overprotective of me because of the cerebral palsy. Instead, they were like, "Ah, fuck it, he'll be fine!"

My brother Greg is the oldest, by ten years. He's easily eight times bigger than me and a stud athlete with a short fuse. He and Dad played Scrabble for money, not much, like a nickel a game, but Greg would get heated. Once, my brother lost and threw a chair through the window. He, too, had trouble communicating with my mother. Greg pretty much ignored me until the day we played football with the neighborhood kids. In the last game, he saw me single-handedly tackle not one but two of his huge friends. I was a super scrawny little fucker, but I would just throw my fourteen-year-old self into their legs and wreck them. Greg told me we could now hang out. A few years ago, he said I wasn't allowed to write any jokes about him or put him in a book. Whoops!

Next up is Jessica, who we call Jess. She's the sibling I emulated the most. She has a wacky sense of humor and is a bit of a loose cannon. She was in love with Prince and never wore shoes unless she had to. She would give me enough details of her grown-up life to keep me interested, but not so much as to be an overly bad influence. Like my mom, Jess was always on the sewing machine, but while my mom stuck to patterns, Jess had her own style, like "what if we cut the sleeves off this dress?"

My sister Emily is the most grounded of all of us, and probably the smartest. We call her The Sniper. She's real quiet, doesn't raise her voice, but when she does pull the trigger, there's no avoiding it. She has a dry sense of humor; for her senior prank, she placed an ad in the newspaper, putting her school up for sale. As the closest sibling, four years my senior, we spent a lot of time together, and we bickered quite a bit. Once, when I was ten, I begged her to tie me to the leg of the baby grand—I considered myself quite the Houdini. She obliged, but I couldn't escape and began crying. Emily ended up getting in trouble despite pointing out I had asked her to do it.

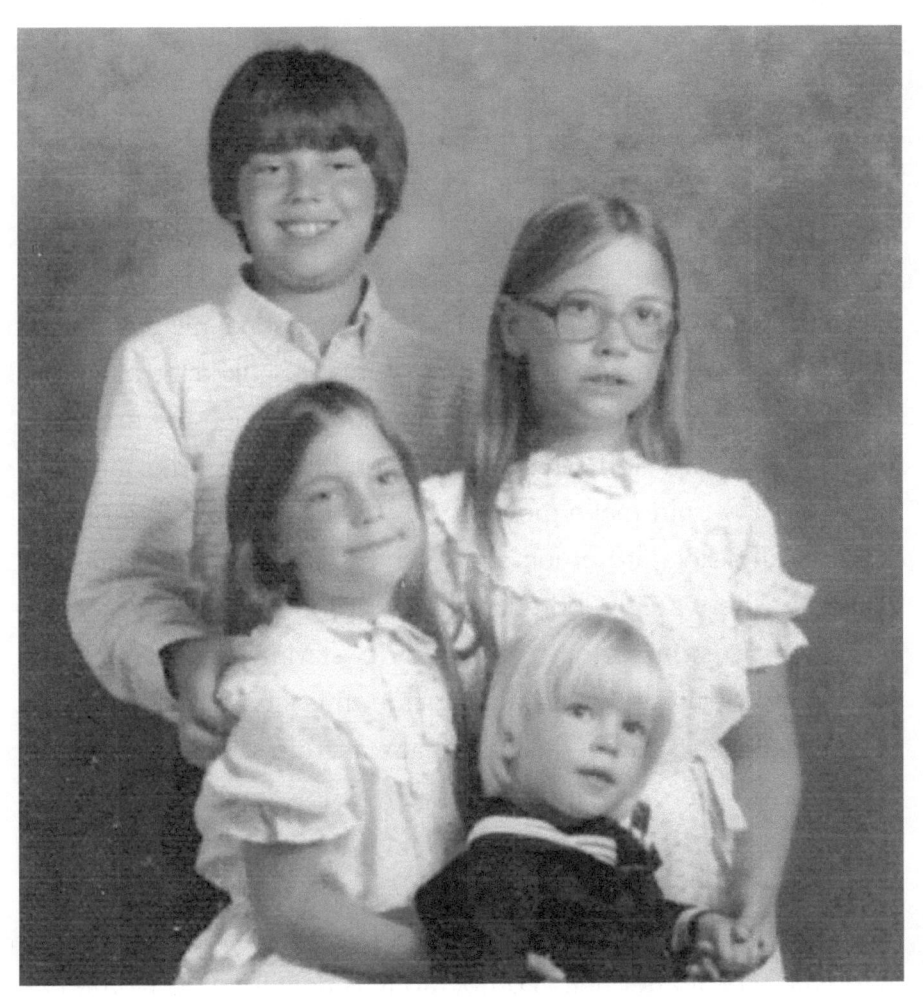

I'm only including this photo because my siblings hate it. Clockwise from top: My brother Greg, sporting his finest homemade haircut, my sister Jess, straight off the set from Little House on the Prairie, some little gay sailor, and my sister Emily, on her way to fall in a well.

My siblings and I all speak English and French, and each of us speaks at least one more bonus language; mine is Wolof. But in my family, I consider my role to be the translator. I can speak to any of my family members on the level they need to be spoken to. I'm the go-between, the mediator for any feuds or just day-to-day communication. I'm sure they would disagree.

I was lucky to have strong women in my life. My sisters, in particular, provided me with their own special type of education. I learned about cruel and dry humor from them. I learned how hard you can push someone's buttons before they snap. They used to dress me up in girl clothes when I was small. "You used to be so cute," they'd tell me. "What happened?" I was their personal rag doll. I don't know if I was too weak to defend myself or if I just liked the attention.

When I was six, our family was walking through the mall, and Jess leaned down and whispered, "Everybody is staring at you." She knew it would make me cry. She was being cruel, but only in the way all sisters are cruel; she wasn't trying to make fun of my disability, she was just bored. Later at home she told me, "Mom said I had to stop saying, 'Everybody is staring at you,' because everybody really is." And that made me cry all over again, because at age six I already knew that was true.

At age seven, my mom received a note at home from my teacher saying she had found bra ads poorly ripped out of the Sears catalog stuffed in my stocking cap. My mom was disappointed, but my sister Jess was furious. She sat me down and made me repeat after her, "Pornography is degrading to women all across the world." About sixty times.

Around age twelve, Emily was verbally tormenting me, and I responded with a rude gesture I had seen at school. I made my left arm stiff, bent my elbow, and started thumping my hand against my chest, moaning, *"Ogh, ogh, ogh."* Emily looked at me, sad and disgusted. Part of her look was knowing this mocking behavior existed in my world. The other part of her look was that I was making fun of myself but didn't know it. I had no idea I was insulting myself until she told me so. I was forcing my left arm to do what my right arm did naturally. I had seen kids do this, but never made the connection to myself. Something clicked in my brain. "Oh fuck, they really do see me like that."

My sisters could get very creative with their teasing. When I was an early tween, they grew very concerned that I hadn't yet had my period. After daily inquiries with hard faces, I too grew concerned.

"You should probably ask Mom about it," Emily said. "And then she'll take you to the doctor."

"And you should start carrying this around with you." Jess handed me a tampon.

In my heart, I knew I couldn't...I didn't...where was I supposed to put that? My big sisters wouldn't lie to me, right? I'm starting to have my doubts. I'm in my forties, and I still haven't blossomed.

When I was sixteen I confided in Jess, "Hey there's a girl in my class I like." I was strongly attracted to the opposite sex, but this girl actually showed *me* some interest, which I thought I would never achieve, due to the palsy.

"She's not a girl," Jess replied. "After a girl has her period, she's a woman."

"Yikes," I said. I didn't know if she had gotten her period yet, but at least I had a tampon to offer her. With furrowed brows, I asked earnestly, "So, by that rationale, when is a boy a man?"

"Twenty-two."

"Well, shit."

16 | *Something To Stare At*

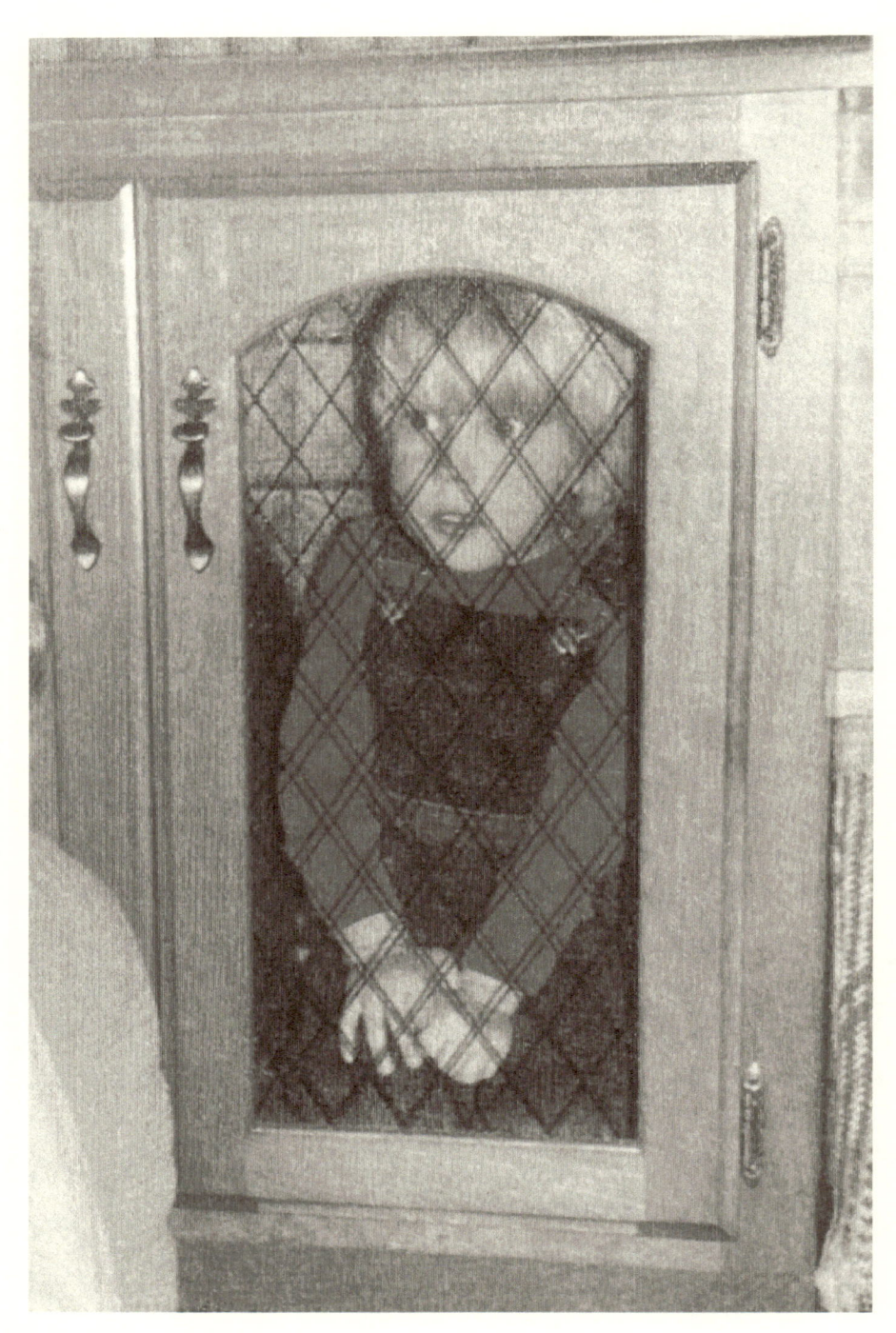

In my special thinking cabinet.

All my siblings went to a prestigious private school, St. Paul Academy. In some sort of social experiment, my parents sent me to Como Park, a much more diverse public school. The trade-off was a shittier education. The truth of the matter is, I was sent to a public school because of my disability.

My first best friend Nick and I met in special-ed preschool. He has a more severe case of cerebral palsy than mine. Nick has the most distinct walk and the biggest heart of any person I know. I could always tell when my friend was coming down the hallway by the *clickety-clack* of his metal crutches. We are the yin and yang of palsy; his lower body is more locked up and rigid than mine, and my upper body is more twisted than his. Also, compared to me, he is a saint.

In special ed, they piled all the mentally and physically disabled kids together in the east wing of the basement. I was treated like I couldn't read, and so I didn't; therefore I couldn't. My writing was a messy scrawl that even I couldn't interpret. Cerebral palsy prevented me from physically writing; being lazy prevented me from reading. I probably could have read at the same level as some of the other kids in my mainstream class, but if the teachers thought I couldn't, why bother to put in the effort?

Despite my difficulties reading, by the fourth grade the teachers knew Nick and I were as clever as, if not more so, than the dumb, able-bodied kids, and thus special ed ended for us. After we were mainstreamed, we stuck together all the way through high school. We still had our cripple perks. The Palsy Duo got to leave class five minutes early so we could have extra time in the hall. We never needed it, but always took it so we could walk by other classrooms to taunt our friends who weren't lucky enough to be disabled.

18 | *Something To Stare At*

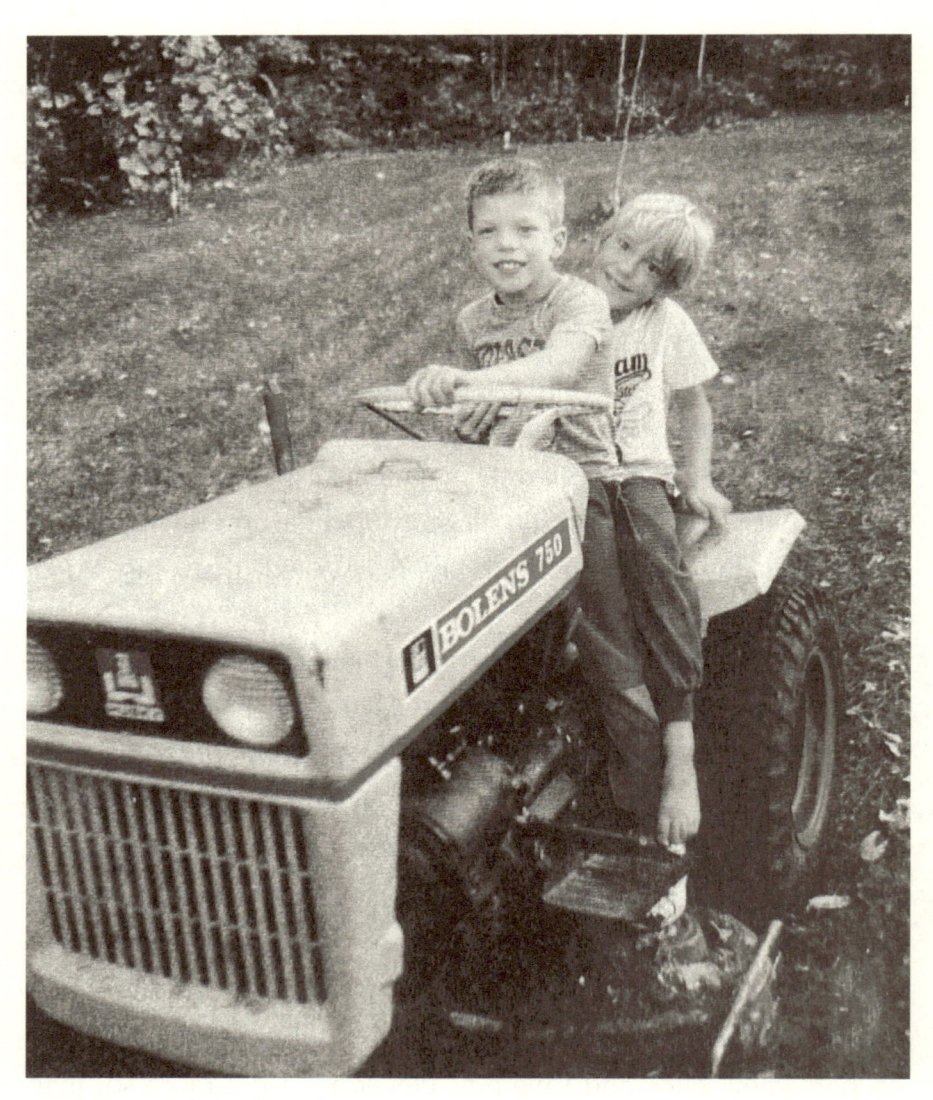

My first joyride with Nick.

If I had gone to a private school, my parents would have had to pay someone to help me with reading and writing. When I was in public junior high, the school provided me with Mrs. Rosa Marie Daniels, a middle-aged Black woman who had just moved from Mississippi. She was the no-nonsense wife of a reverend and came to school every day dressed like she was going to church. She took

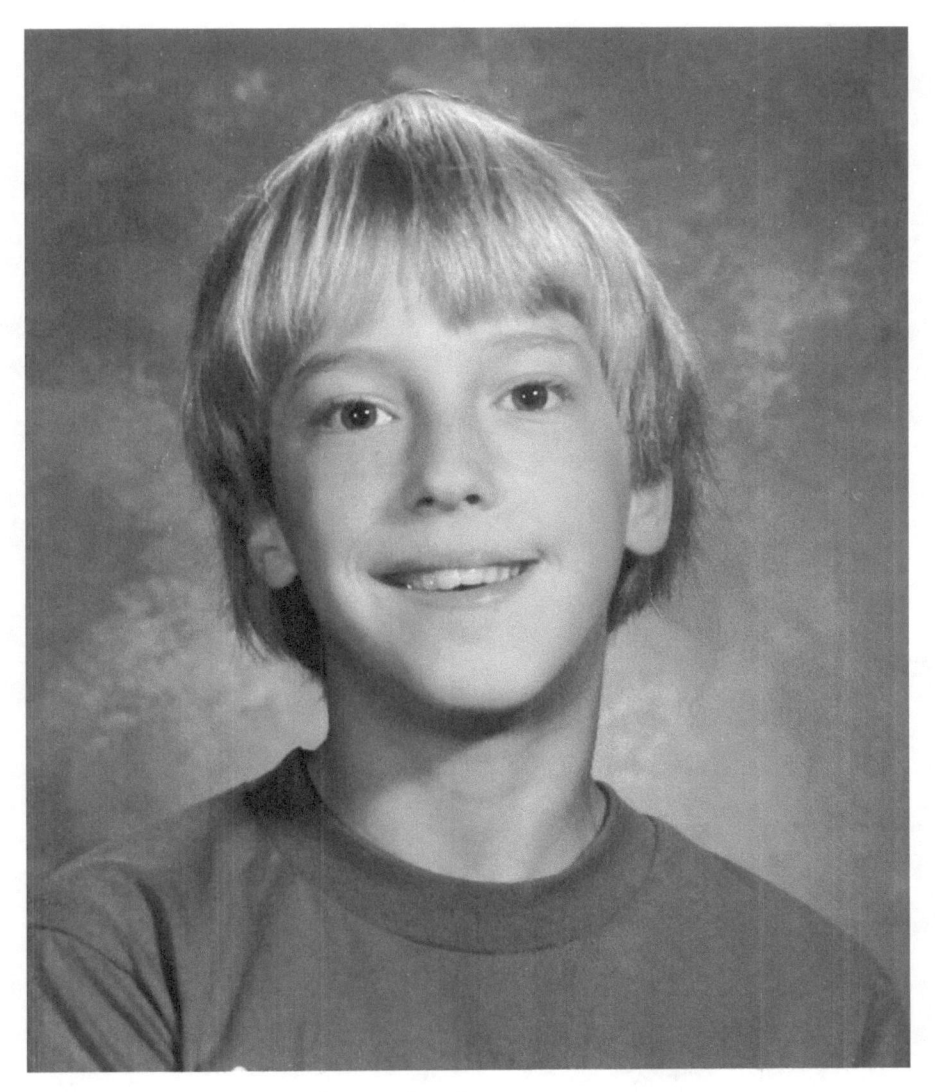

Hard to believe I got so hairy after this.

notes for me, wrote out my assignments, and for tests, she and I went to a separate room and I dictated my answers to her.

Mrs. Daniels had those big, fake, Lee press-on nails that she painted in class. The stink of the polish was strong, but the teachers never said anything because they were as intimidated by her as I was. One day, I heard her rhythmically drumming those big, long nails on the desk, and I asked, "Are you bored?"

"Yeah, I am," she snapped. "I've already went to school. Now turn around and pay attention, boy!"

Hearing that was strangely eye-opening for me. Of course she was bored. What a horrible job, following my dumb ass around every day. It made me realize how patient Mrs. Daniels could be.

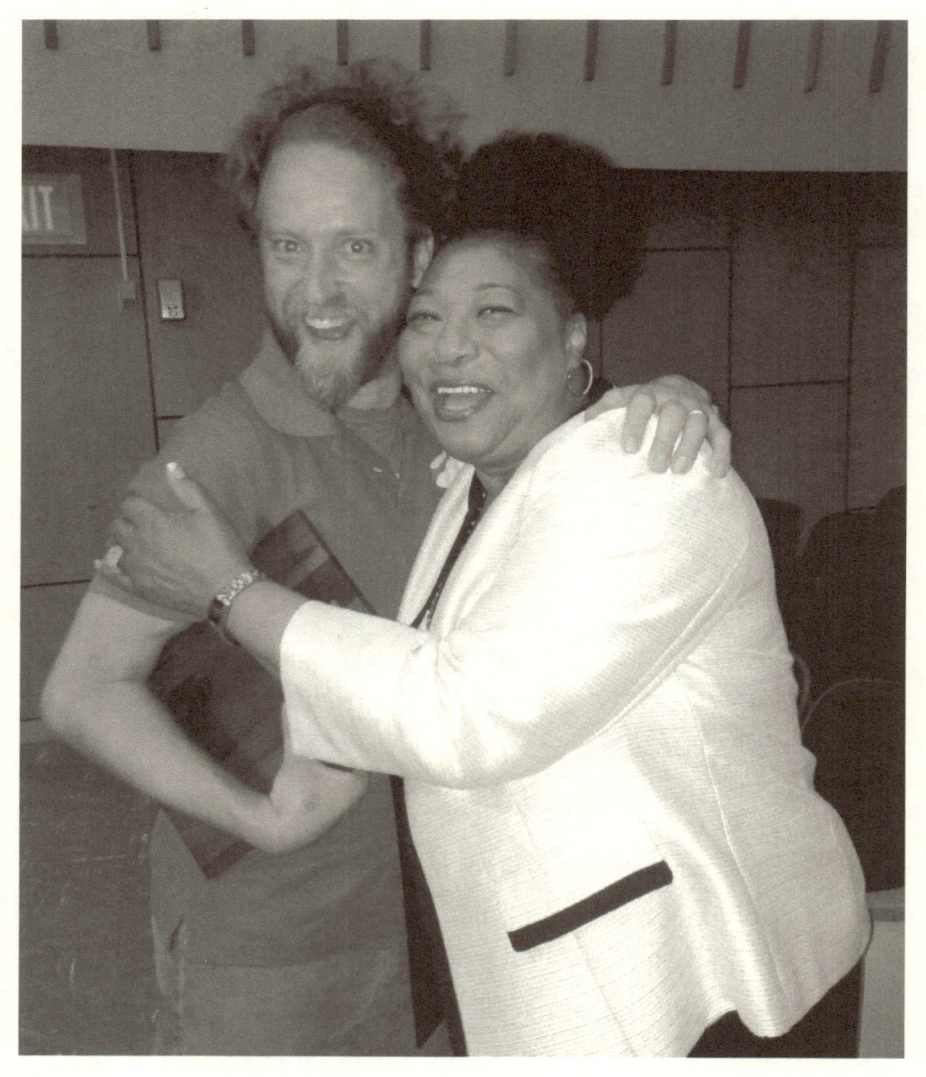

The woman, the myth, the legend: Mrs. Daniels. A surprise reunion in 2007.

Once, in seventh-grade French class, we had a substitute teacher named Madame Hoover. A sub is usually cause for celebration, but Madame Hoover took an instant liking to me. Like I was a new channel of inspiration porn.

She could tell I had palsy, because you can tell I have palsy, and the presence of Mrs. Daniels was a bit of a tell. Madame Hoover started asking overly simple questions about my day-to-day life. "Whyyy diiid youuu chooose Freeench claaass?" When she addressed me, she spoke louder and slower, with exaggerated hand gestures.

My friends and I snickered in the back of the classroom.

"This lady's a real freak," I whispered to my friend Marney.

Madame Hoover was in mid-sentence about Napoleon when she turned to me. "Josh, I haaave a speeecial liiittle friennnd juuust liiike youuu. Youuu aaare sooo couraaageous. And youuu aaare both sooo inspiraaationaaal."

The silence that followed was like being underwater and lasted longer than I could possibly hold my breath. I caught my tongue and squelched my reaction to get up and punch her. I slipped into the play-along game. "Reaaally?" I said, slowing the cadence of my speech to match her expectations. "He must be suuuper patient to have a friend like youuu." My classmates barely concealed their amusement. Mrs. Daniels was painting her nails, silently approving my performance.

After twenty minutes of back-and-forth, it was so painful that Marney finally re-directed Madame Hoover's attention to the lesson at hand. "Hey, don't we have a project we're supposed to be doing?" It was only a one-hour class, and this moron had spent more than half of it on me. I figured I'd paid my karmic dues, and she'd leave me alone for the rest of the period.

"Yes. We'll be making posters about the Eiffel Tower," said Madame Hoover. So we got our art supplies: scissors, tag board, and markers. I was up front, getting the markers from the teacher's table, and Madame Hoover said even slower this time, "Jooosh caaan youuu haaand meee the oooorange maaarker? The ooorange maaarker?"

I gave the class a little wink and handed Madame Hoover a purple marker.

In the early fall, there were open tryouts for the school's soccer team. Some of my classmates were pretty big soccer studs, and they encouraged me to try out. This was my first time staying after school for any reason. I felt like a big kid, even if it took me twenty minutes to wrestle on my never-been-worn soccer socks and muster up the courage to ask one of my potential teammates to tie my shoes for me.

The first day, we did some light drills and technical work. I was certainly not the best player on the field, but I was also not the worst. It was not my first time around a soccer ball, but it was my first time going out for a team. Since I was born in Cameroon, my family is a strong supporter of their national team, the Indomitable Lions. All my siblings played the game, and both my sisters went to state with their fancy private high school teams.

On the second day, we scrimmaged as the Minnesota fall was leaning toward winter. I didn't score, but I didn't play like shit either. It was fun hanging out with the guys after practice, and I had a blast making everybody laugh, on and off the field.

The third day, I was warming up with the team, and the coach walked up to me.

"Hi Coach!" I said with a smile.

"What are you doing here?" Before I could answer, he added, "Didn't you get the letter for your parents? It had your refund check for your tryout."

"No," I murmured, as I recalled the letter the teacher had handed me in third hour. It was addressed to my parents, so I didn't open it.

"I've selected my team," he said.

As I fought back tears, I looked onto the field and had the harsh revelation that the kids I thought I was better than weren't there either. I had to retrieve my soccer ball from the boys who made the team.

Now crying, I made my way off the field to a big oak tree, hopefully out of earshot. I sat there fighting to take off my stupid socks and feeling bad for myself. Part of me worried that my period could be coming on.

The coach blew the whistle, and the chosen team gathered around him. I stayed there the entire practice, watching. It was before cell phones, and my mom wasn't picking me up until after practice. Even though the experience didn't stop me from loving the game, it prevented me from feeling good enough about myself to try out for any team for years.

HIGH SCHOOL

High school was a weird popularity contest. People generally stuck to their cliques, but then there was Hector Caballero. He looked just like Ponch from the American television series *CHiPs*. He was in my homeroom freshman year and quickly became my second best friend after Nick. He was outspoken and unafraid, even of Mrs. Daniels.

My family fell in love with Hector. I would come home to find him sitting at the piano with my dad, belting out show tunes. My dad often playfully remarked that Hector was the son he always wanted. And of course my sisters loved Hector's quick, sick sense of humor.

We were a peculiar combo, because Hector was a devout Catholic and staunch Republican, and I was cool. Hector was the first person I met who was nonstop funny, and I soon realized I

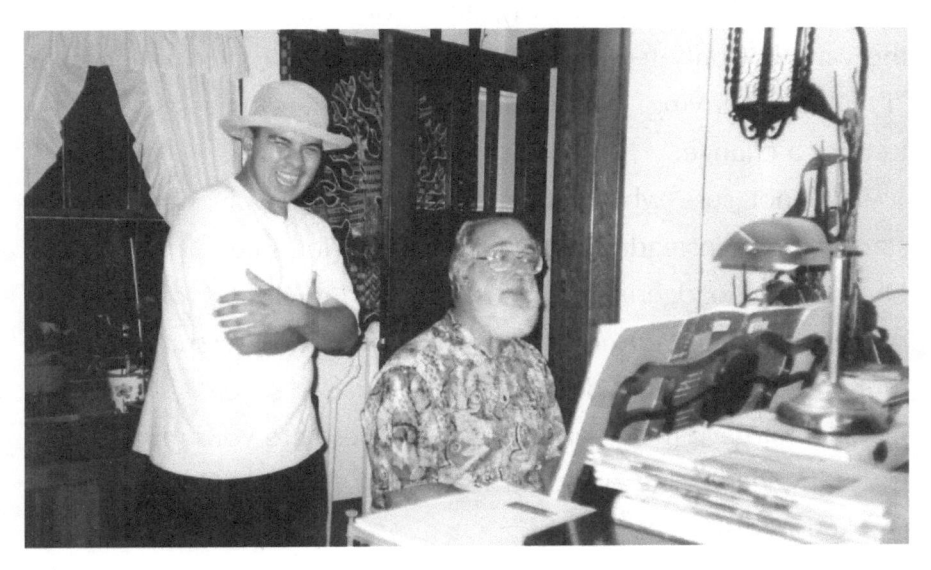

My father and his real son, Hector.

could match him comedically. My mom and dad always said that when Hector and I were together, no one else had a clue what we were laughing at. It's our own language, and it's painfully funny.

A defining milestone in our friendship came when Hector offered to give me a ride home from school. I had ridden the bus my whole life, and now, here was a friend willing to go out of his way to drive me in his very own car, a beat-to-shit red Camaro. Every tire was a different size and brand. There were no functioning seat belts. The doors were so long and heavy I had to lean half my body out, anchor my feet under the dashboard, grab the handle with both hands, and use all my strength to slam the clunky door. There were flecks of cigarette ash floating all over the hot, black interior. The car looked like it had been through a Holy War.

He would eventually destroy that car with a crowbar in a fit of jealous rage.

One night on the freeway, after hours of aimlessly driving in the way that only teenagers can do, Hector abruptly pulled over. "I'm sick of driving. We're not going anywhere unless you take a turn for a change."

I'm not sure why Hector thought the freeway was the best starting point instead of a desolate parking lot. I kept refusing, and Hector kept badgering. *Why is he offering up his most prized possession to certain disaster?* But the more he pressured me, the more I thought I could do it. Finally, we traded seats.

Hector gave me a vague tutorial: "These are your mirrors. Gas is on the right." He punched in the car lighter. "Gonna need a smoke for this."

I touched my shaking foot to the gas pedal with what I

thought was a cautious amount of pressure, and the Camaro's big engine roared to life. We lunged forward onto the freeway as the tires spat gravel out behind us.

"Go with the flow," Hector shouted over the roar of the wind. "And blinkers are optional."

My eyes bugged out of their sockets. I was white-knuckling the wheel with my left hand as my right arm danced around the car and occasionally landed on the cold steering wheel.

"Usually, I'd encourage people to keep two hands on the wheel." Hector laughed, dodging my flailing arm to light his cigarette.

After a few miles, I pulled off at an exit ramp and stopped the car. "I'm sick of driving," I said. "We're not going anywhere unless you take the wheel."

Hector flicked his cigarette butt out the window, radiating joy despite the obvious peril he had put himself in. He stopped laughing just long enough to light another cigarette, then took over driving.

This was not only a landmark in my life as my first time behind the wheel, but another defining moment in my friendship with Hector. Sure, he was clearly batshit crazy, but he also treated me in an able-bodied way, even if it was grossly irresponsible.

Hector never let me drive his car again. I've driven four times in my life since then, and I've been in two minor accidents. Fifth time's the charm.

Our homeroom teacher was directing the senior class production of *The Man Who Came to Dinner*. I knew Hector would have one of the leads. The more I heard kids talking about the play, the more exciting it seemed. My teacher could tell I was curious.

"Josh, you should really audition," she said. "I have the perfect role for you, and you would definitely have a unique stage presence."

"That'd be the only way you'll come to one of my performances," Hector said, handing Mrs. Daniels a piece of gum as she laughed and seconded the encouragement.

I was hesitant, to say the least. I thought it would be fun, but auditioning was more terrifying than driving Hector's car. I had never been onstage before, and the last time I had tried out for something—the soccer team—I was devastated. Just walking down the high school hallways felt like a daily audition, putting myself on display for the judgment of my pimply peers. The school play was open to the whole world.

And I did it.

My audition was a monologue about a missing sock. I flubbed a few words, but my timing was good. My only feedback was a quiet thank you, and I left the room uncertain of how I had performed. The next day, the teacher surprised me with the part and, for some reason, felt obligated to tell me that I was the only one to even audition for that role. They just needed a warm body, and my acting was apparently just better than a corpse.

I was happy to take on my new role as Sandy, the lovable labor union worker, with lovably limited dialogue. Hector had landed the role of Banjo, a rascally character that my own father had played in his high school days. I took to calling them Banjo and Banjo. "Hey Banjo and Banjo, can you keep it down over there? I'm trying to watch *Garfield*!"

It wasn't until rehearsals and improv games that I realized how funny Hector and I really were together. The quick rapport we had built over years of verbal fencing made us the highlight of every improv game. We were the fun ones, the funny guys.

I loved the fear and adrenaline of the improv games and learning to trust my instincts to say the right thing at the right time. I liked it much more than the scripted dialogue, and it turned out I had a knack for it. I found I could be funny and quick with anyone, not just Hector, and I loved building a scene out of my imagination.

After many months of practice, it was finally opening night. When it was my cue, I was supposed to come out of the kitchen door for my big debut. Apparently there was some concern that I was not going to do this, so Allison, my fellow student and stage director who I had a crush on, stood by me with a calm hand on my shoulder, ready to forcibly shove me out onstage. I took a deep breath and wiped my sweaty, shaky hands on my costume. My cue came, and I stepped out.

My scene went by in a blur. When I left the stage, Allison gave me a big hug and a kiss on the cheek. "You did great! I'm so proud of you."

It was my first kiss. I was a bit confused. *Does everybody get a kiss after their scene?* Allison became my first girlfriend, and we dated for a whole week.

Now I had a new motivation. From there on out, I equated performing with the chance of getting more kisses. I didn't think most thespians got into acting to get girls, but maybe this was my way in. Plus, working in theater was validating. I already had the ability to make friends and strangers laugh, but the theater made it seem like a viable undertaking to pursue on a bigger scale.

Even though being onstage was terrifying for me, it became fiercely addictive. I loved the exhilarating rush of being in front of people and getting them to react at the appropriate point, and then the wash of relief once it was over, as well as overcoming something I was petrified of.

After surviving a successful run of *The Man Who Came to Dinner*, one of the actors threw a low-key cast party at their parents' house. It was a nice house, in a nice neighborhood, on a hill overlooking the seminary. Because we were theater dweebs, there was no alcohol. Instead, we were verbally one-upping each other in the basement.

The doorbell rang.

When we went outside, it was dusk, and all the gigantic maple trees were draped in toilet paper. We could see an idling minivan at the bottom of the hill, admiring their work from the seminary parking lot.

In defense of thespians everywhere, the entire cast gave chase down the hill and made a move to block the only exit to the parking lot. Hector led the charge with a war cry. I picked up a large tree branch, others had rocks. We were out for blood. How dare they interrupt our boring-ass party!

As we reached the exit, the culprits punched the gas, and I had to dive out of the way to not get hit. Some kids ran uselessly after them down the street while Hector and I sprinted up the hill to his Camaro. We jumped in, and he had the car moving before I was able to close the door.

We chased them through the neighborhood as they tried to flee the scene, doing things like putting on their left blinker, and then abruptly turning right. Unfortunately for them, Hector didn't believe in blinkers.

They had a pretty good lead, and Hector mysteriously stopped at a red light. When the light changed, Hector gunned it toward the freeway entrance.

"No, they went down the frontage road!" I shouted as we merged into speeding traffic.

"I know," Hector said as he calmly lit a cigarette and popped *Guys and Dolls* into the cassette player.

As "Luck Be a Lady" started up, I looked out my window, down the embankment at the minivan. I could finally see the chubby-cheeked driver and his friends, who I recognized from school. The minivan slowed to stay parallel to us as they smiled and gloated, thinking they had given us the slip.

"I'll show you luck, lady!" Hector screamed as he jammed the hot Camaro down the steep embankment, angling the shuddering car toward the broad side of the now accelerating minivan. The driver's expression went from smug to terrified, as he realized that the person chasing him was far more dedicated to this game than he was. I shared his terror.

Hector didn't give a shit. He was going to ram them. But their old minivan was more nimble than our shitty Camaro. They pulled away into the warehouse district. We followed them into a cul-de-sac, believing them cornered, but we underestimated the amazing turning radius of their vehicle.

By the time Hector executed a four-point turn, they were out of sight, fleeing in the direction from where we had come. As we rounded a corner, we saw them in the distance, getting on the freeway ramp, headed in our direction. I didn't have to look at Hector to know where this was going. He revved the engine, hurtled down the frontage road, and swerved back up the embankment. This maneuver caused the cassettes on the dashboard to slide toward the open window on my side.

"My Fiddler!" Hector screamed as they slid out of his reach. I made no attempt to stop them, and they flew out the window.

Hector's trajectory was almost perfect, and we bounced back onto the freeway, just missing the minivan. We were greeted with oncoming headlights and horns, which Hector remedied with a life-saving U-turn.

It was too late. They had vanished into the night's traffic. We drove around for another forty minutes, looking for them. Hector even had the balls to stop a police cruiser and ask if they'd seen some White boys causing trouble.

My two best friends were the best of enemies. Without me as their common denominator, Nick and Hector probably would have killed each other. Nick's stiff body could never move fast enough for Hector's liking. One time at Nick's house, Hector pushed Nick down to help him put his shoes on when we were getting ready to go out.

"Can't you put these on any faster? Jesus Christ!" Hector said, crouching at Nick's feet.

"Hector!" I cut in.

"Shut up, we're going to be late!" Hector yelled, throwing Nick's coat at him as Nick was trying to stand up.

"For what? Taco Bell?" I retorted in Nick's defense. Nick could never tell Hector to fuck off in a way that Hector could hear it.

We searched for entertainment after school in the Twin Cities, but there was never enough to keep us occupied. We usually ended up at the mall, even though none of us had any money to spend. It was a good place to check out the ladies. Picture us: two cripples and a Mexican trying to pick up chicks. I'm not saying being Mexican is a disability, but being a Republican Mexican is.

Now, it's hard enough to get positive female attention when

you are one disabled person, but when you are in a small herd of cripples, it makes it damn near impossible. I often thought people must think Hector is our caretaker, and one day, a wicked idea struck me.

Hector was being his usual dickish self, stepping up the pace and hurrying Nick just to be mean.

"We don't have anywhere to be," Nick said, deliberately slowing down.

Once Hector was out of earshot, I said to Nick, "He wants handicaps...he's gonna get handicaps." I could tell by Nick's labored, palsy smile that he totally understood.

"Hector, can you come here a minute?" I yelled.

"What do you want?" he snapped as he brazenly strolled back toward us.

"Hector! You not good caretaker!" I shouted, distorting my face and my body into a cripply collage.

"*N-n-n-yaaagh*, you hit us! Don't hit!" Nick chimed in.

Hector's normally unflappable demeanor was instantly shattered. "What the fuck?" he said, almost to himself.

A small crowd was forming, pretty girls and all.

"*N-n-n-yaaagh!*" With this cry, I produced a large strand of drool. I could see the whole fight-or-flight process go through Hector's head. What were his options? Either assault two disabled kids in front of a now concerned and growing audience, or flee in uncharacteristic cowardice. He chose the latter.

Hector turned and ran, muttering curses under his breath. I took off after him, gleeful to be chasing him for once. I kept fifteen paces behind, running like a cross between a monkey and a paraplegic, squealing with delight at the top of my lungs, "*N-n-n-yaaagh!*"

Twenty paces behind me, Nick was running at his full speed, shouting, "*Gah-gah*, don't leave me behind again! *Gah-gah!*"

We ran through the mall like this, with the *clickety-clack* of Nick's arm crutches echoing us all the way back to the parking lot where Hector was clearly rushing to leave us but fumbling with his keys, like he himself was now stricken with palsy.

Nick and I laughed the whole ride home as Hector berated us with empty threats. "If you two cockbags ever pull that shit again, I'll never drive you anywhere!"

Deep down, I knew Hector had to respect our prank. It was a good dose of his own medicine. Of course, it didn't change his behavior at all, but at least he now knew what Nick and I were capable of.

I had nine friends that lived on my block, and they all lived in the same house. They were the Nguyen siblings. Since I was old enough to walk (like, when I was seven), we spent our days running back and forth between our houses. My friends wanted to come to my house because we had lots of food and toys. I wanted to go to their house, because it was more dangerous; with twelve kids, there was no way their parents could be everywhere at once.

The Nguyen siblings treated me like number thirteen, just another one of the crew. Whenever I fell, the herd would stop running, come back and dust off their broken White brother, and we would continue the adventure. Our favorite pastime was descending on the neighbors' gardens like a plague of locusts to eat their fruits and vegetables.

"You gooks get out of my garden!" someone yelled. I was honored to be insulted alongside them. After that, one of the younger brothers always called me Gook.

There was no problem the thirteen of us couldn't solve.

One bright summer day, all of us kids were out in the Nguyen's front yard playing whatever we played. I was eight or nine at the time. There was an older White boy across the street who we all called Bobby the Brain, even though he was a racist dumbass. He would go out of his way to be mean to us. On this particular day, he kept shining a little makeup mirror across the street, catching the sun and hitting us in the eyes. All the siblings huddled together and had a quick conference in Vietnamese. One brother opened the front door, and they all filed into the house, leaving me in the yard.

Bobby the Brain and I were left staring at each other, then he directed his mirror at me. I could tell he was as curious about what they were up to as I was, although I was sure it wasn't going to end well for old Bobby.

We didn't have to wait long.

I heard an upstairs window slide open. My crew had grabbed a huge mirror from the top of an armoire and were laboriously dragging it onto the roof like a team of angry ants. They positioned the mirror to reflect the sun down on Bobby, 800 times the strength of his puny mirror, strong enough to melt his car. Shielding his face, Bobby the Brain retreated inside as I laughed and cheered, furthering his humiliation. When you messed with one of us, you messed with all of us. I was proud of my tribe.

()()()

Being born in Cameroon, I felt a strong connection to Africa, even though I was just a little guy when we left. I remember watching National Geographic shows and feeling a strong pull every time anything about Africa came on. It was my ace in the hole talking point, and I used it to deflect attention away from the palsy. They'd say, "You're different," and I'd say, "I am different. I was born in Africa. You've never been out of the state."

It was a dream come true when my parents told me we were moving to Senegal for a year. I was fifteen. This time my dad was going to be teaching American literature at the University of Saint Louis in the north of Senegal, up along the mighty Senegal River. My dear friend Klaus was tagging along. He was also born in Africa, and his parents had worked as Lutheran missionaries in Madagascar. Since all of my siblings were off in college or living on their own, my parents wanted to bring someone who could keep up with me and keep me occupied.

One of my earliest memories of Klaus is when we stole his older brother's tape of Eddie Murphy's comedy album and secretly listened to it under a blanket in the basement. Eddie said the term "rubber penis," and it broke us. Just the utterance of it would send us into tears of laughter and pain-inducing giggles for years to come.

We would both be home-schooled by my mother. I was ecstatic about getting away from traditional school, from the hardships of being mainstreamed as a disabled person. I would miss Nick and Hector, and I wondered what Mrs. Daniels would do without me; but I saw the opportunity as a respite, something new to talk about when I returned to the States.

My father told us we should pick a Senegalese name, or someone in Senegal would pick one for us or call us *toubab* which means White person. My sister Emily (who would be joining us there later) and I looked through the list of first and last names. I settled on Babacar Djot. I wanted her to pick Adji Badji or Poopette, but she went with Aminata.

Our journey would take us from Minneapolis to Paris to Nouakchott, the capital of Mauritania, then finally landing in Dakar. We'd have a day in Dakar before driving north to Saint Louis. On the first leg of our journey, I sat next to Klaus, with my parents sitting a few rows back. There was no drinking age on transatlantic flights, so it was time to try out my high school French. *"Vin rouge,"* I told the stewardess confidently.

Without hesitation, she handed us teenager-sized bottles of Merlot. I drank mine straight from the bottle, cutting out the flimsy, plastic cup middleman.

We had a five-hour layover in Paris—I hadn't been there since I was a dying baby. We didn't have enough time to leave the airport, only enough to wander around, try out more of my freshman French, and annoy the Parisians, which wasn't hard.

"Où se trouvent les toilettes?" I said, standing directly in front of the men's room. I found my French flowed better on a couple of red wines.

The flight to Nouakchott was five-and-a-half hours. Gliding 37,000 feet above the Sahara desert, there was nothing but a sand ocean in every direction. I drank on that flight, too. I was on my first but far from last international bender.

The layover in Nouakchott was a blur. The final leg to Dakar was quick and a time to celebrate with a little bottle of champagne. What I didn't anticipate was the oncoming rollercoaster ride—the bubbles of champagne fighting with the vin rouge. The wicked turbulence made the plane slam down, and with that, the bender ended in the little white bag that was conveniently provided in the seat pocket in front of me.

As we gathered our belongings to exit, I still had the

disgusting, party-filled paper bag in my right hand. I didn't know what to do with it. I looked around the plane and saw my parents. They didn't acknowledge my greenish hue or the bag of vomit. They looked tired. I pulled my backpack out from under the seat in front of me and softball-pitched the barf bag in its place.

On the tarmac, it was dark. Smells were all I had to give me a hint of what the daylight would bring. A warm, muggy breeze, soaked with everything Africa, hit me in the face. It was like being in a terrarium. The air smelled like fruit and garbage with a hint of piss and woodsmoke.

It felt good to be back.

The next morning, Klaus and I were restless to see as much Africa as possible, so my dad walked us to the beach. *The ocean must be close, I can smell it.* It turned out to be a long walk to the water. As the three of us picked our way toward the beach, every taxi that passed would honk and slow down, taking note of my awkward gait. I could feel them fixate on me; they had probably never seen a disabled White person before and thought I must need a taxi.

My dad repeatedly turned down the drivers in Wolof, the language of Senegal and of some of its neighbors. We kept walking. Every bush and tree had some new, exciting bird in it; every leaf had a different bug. Then, caught in the light, I saw a spider the size of a lemon, colored like a bumblebee, floating on its yellow web, each strand as thick and strong as dental floss.

The roar of the ocean called my attention away from the giant spider. I was taking in this new world like a curious toddler, as though I was resuming my life in Africa after being born here. The beach was busy for an early morning. A man was renting boogie boards at a little kiosk and my dad agreed to rent one for us. Klaus and I took turns, each getting five tries to ride a wave.

I went first, without much success. I did manage to get rolled across the punishing ocean floor by a big wave, and spitting up sandy saltwater was already better than whatever I'd be doing back on the frozen plains of Minnesota. I smiled, thinking of Nick and Hector, miserably sitting at their desks at school. I hoped Hector was taking it easy on Nick without me there to referee.

Klaus went next, and he immediately had the hang of it. Four out of his five rides were smooth. I don't think he even got his tight, curly blond hair wet.

We kept at it for an hour or so. I had the board when Klaus yelled that his leg was hurt and that he needed to get out of the water. There was a wavy, red stripe wrapping around his inner thigh. A dreadlocked man saw Klaus limping out of the water and came over to offer assistance. Or I might have been the one who drew his attention first. I would have been limping, too.

The man studied us with his brilliant eyes. He saw the mark on Klaus's leg and said, "Jellyfish," in English, then moved calmly to the lifeguard station and grabbed a bottle of salve. The man spoke more to us in Wolof. Even though we couldn't understand what he was saying, we understood what he was doing. His mellowness rubbed off on Klaus.

Klaus never cried, though it looked so painful. I know I would have cried.

At some point, my dad noticed us and tore himself away from his crossword puzzle. He spoke to the man in a mix of French and Wolof. The man was moving the whole time, his calmness never altered. As he worked the salve into Klaus's leg, he assured my dad he would be fine. Then he focused his attention on me, who looked to be the one who needed more permanent assistance. The way he was treating me and my fidgety body, it was like he was interviewing for a job as my caretaker. Without asking, he sat me down and brushed the wet sand off my feet, putting my socks on, leaving injured Klaus to dress himself. He seemed to be trying to negotiate a deal with my dad.

"We won't be staying in Dakar," my dad said. "We're headed to Saint Louis later this afternoon."

On the walk back, the guy followed us halfway to our hotel, pleading his case. "I can go to Saint Louis!"

By now, Klaus was shaking more than I was. My dad told us, "Never turn your back on the ocean," which is good advice, but a little late for Klaus.

The liaison from the university in Saint Louis said he'd pick us up at one o'clock. He showed up at three thirty.

My dad explained to me, "This is what we call 'Africa time.'" He added, "If you want to meet somebody at a certain time, always tell them two hours earlier."

The man from the university showed up in a loud embroidered shirt, much like the ones my dad always wore. My dad did the introductions in French, Wolof, and English so we could all understand. We loaded our bags onto the roof rack of the three-row station wagon and headed north.

We left Dakar, the westernmost tip of Africa, and drove almost to the border of Mauritania. The car ride was its own introduction to Senegal: beautiful high-cheek-boned women carrying mounds of produce on their heads, donkey carts next to boxy Mercedes, dark faces with darker aviator glasses, countless free-roaming chickens, long-horned cattle with protruding hip bones, purple and blue butterflies, and vibrant birds. I was looking for monkeys, but I only saw one sad baboon chained to a tree.

As we approached Saint Louis, the sky was dark, and all we could see were the city's lights. We had to drive over a long bridge spanning the Senegal River, because the city was a large rectangular island in the middle of the dark water. We rode through the blocks of French colonial architecture to the Flamingo Restaurant. We devoured *brochettes*—hunks of skewered goat meat in the spiciest sauce I've ever had—served with rice. It was new to me, and it was delicious.

After dinner and a short walking tour, the driver took us back across the long bridge toward our new home. The university was ten miles outside of city center. A large unit of young, serious men in dark camouflage were marching across the bridge from the opposite direction.

"Soldiers in training," said the driver.

The recruits could only be seen when they passed under the streetlights, and then they were gone. Nobody in the car said anything, but my mom's body language was uneasy.

I was tired. The jet lag had set in, the meat had set in, and the rest of the ride was a drowsy haze. The thrill of what was to come was all that kept me awake.

At the entrance to the university, there was a security checkpoint with a gate. The driver told the guard, *"C'est le nouveau professeur."*

We could see the silhouette of the main campus buildings up ahead. Gnarled trees lined the road on either side. Every fourth or fifth streetlight was off, giving the campus a deserted atmosphere. It was another ten minutes past the gate before we pulled into the loop of all the foreign professors' houses. The yards were big, hundreds of feet between each fence. Our house stood in an expanse of sand and snarly acacia trees.

I was reinvigorated by the excitement of exploring our new home. The yard was huge compared to our lot back in the States. The first thing I noticed were the four meticulously trimmed, perfectly round and symmetrical bushes in the yard. The house was one sprawling ground floor with a flat roof, much wider than my home in Minnesota.

There were no lights on at the house, and my father fumbled with the keys. In the shadows, I saw a peculiarly straight stick. I leaned in closer and realized it was a nicely worn watchman's billy club. The bags in my hands didn't allow me to snatch it up, but I turned to Klaus and said, "I got dibs on that!"

Before Klaus could see what I was talking about, the door was flung open, and we hurried in, weary travelers eager to be at our final stop. It took a while to find the lights. When we finally did, we were standing in a dark-red tiled foyer. And we were not alone. We were greeted by thumb-sized creatures, scattering in all directions. *Are these mice?* They started zig-zagging up the wall. One of them stopped where the wall meets the floor, and I saw legs—six of them. We were surrounded by huge cockroaches. Their shells were almond-shaped, a cold magenta color. My family froze.

The driver laughed nervously, *"Cafard."*

I killed the first one accidentally. It was desperately looking for a shadowy place to hide, and my palsy reflex had me on my tiptoes. The roach made the poor choice to hide under my shoe. I didn't want to step on it, but I got so scared that I lost my balance, and my foot snapped down. There was a moment of resistance, and then it made three separate sickening pops, echoing through the expanse of our new home.

After that initial kill, we all threw our bags down and ran around turning on lights, stomping and swatting. Klaus grabbed one of his newly acquired flip-flops out of his bag, and I ran for my new billy club. My dad frantically pointed out lurking cockroaches for Klaus and me to seek and destroy. These were no one-hit roaches. Klaus would stun them with his flip-flop, and I would crush them with my billy club. Each time I got one, it popped like a gut-filled balloon. There was always an antenna or a leg still twitching.

By the time my mom put clean sheets on all our mattresses, the roach death toll was in the high teens. Despite the exhilaration of my first roach showdown, I succumbed to jet lag. I told myself the sooner I go to sleep, the sooner I wake up and begin my adventure in Africa. I laid my billy club on the nightstand and dreamed of how I'd use it in the morning.

I didn't make it until morning. I awoke to a presence on my body, followed by a sharp pinch through my recently acquired chest hair. That set off the palsy mousetrap. I smacked at the source of the pain and lunged for the light. To my horror, I found a huge roach, the size of a lighter, sitting statuesquely on my bed in a proud pose.

As I edged for my new love, the billy club, I wondered how the roach had ventured so far on my body without waking me. Club in hand, I swung down hard. My errant strike turned the bed into a roach trampoline, launching the bug straight up above my head. I spastically swung two more times on the way down, but whiffed. The roach stuck its landing like a tiny, gross gymnast.

The roach appeared to be enjoying our little game and was

going for gold. Upon dismounting, the roach unfolded its wings with a terrifying click and jetted straight for my face. I swung wildly and finally connected; the sound was like a seashell hitting the floor. The roach, totally unharmed, scurried under the bed to wait for its score. With a serial killer's resolve, I dropped to my hands and knees in hot pursuit. The roach effortlessly jumped up into the box spring, and I craned my neck to watch it run upside down across the boards. Perfect 10.

My mom came in to find me in my boxers on my belly, half under the bed, thumping loudly at the roach, which remained out of reach.

I looked up, wild-eyed. "Get your war paint."

I went back to sleep defeated and slept until dawn, which was when the birds woke me up with their rude, alien singing, squawking, and yelling. I put on my shorts and grabbed my billy club, hoping to catch my new nocturnal nemesis sleeping in the open, but he was nowhere to be found, safely tucked away in his roach hotel. I headed outside, eager to see what my new avian alarm clock looked like.

My mom was doing the heavy lifting of unpacking and organizing the kitchen, while my dad was sipping black coffee and brushing up on his Wolof. He turned from his book long enough to warn me, "Better put on some shoes. Who knows what kind of worms you can get?"

Ignoring him outright, I ran out the front door into the African sun. I was used to running everywhere barefoot. The neighbors back home told me I was the first kid to take my shoes off in the spring, and the last to put them on in the Minnesota winter.

Out past our fence there was a small pack of feral dogs

studying me from the shade of an acacia tree in the center of the housing loop. The sidewalk was already surprisingly hot and, to escape the burning concrete, I jumped toward the shade of one of the four spherical bushes in my new yard. As I hit the sand, I was met with excruciating pain in both feet. I lost my balance and fell backward onto the smoldering sidewalk. My soles were completely covered with what looked like little brown seed pods. I frantically tried to brush them off, and the sharp pain transferred to my hand—little heartless burrs with spikes sticking in every direction.

Klaus came out behind me. "What are you doing?"

"Don't go in the sand!" I shrieked.

Klaus stayed put; he wasn't taking any chances after the jellyfish.

I pulled the burrs out one at a time, then Klaus plucked them out of my fingers. We had to be painstakingly careful (emphasis on pain) so a spine wouldn't break off and stick in my finger or foot. We must have pulled eighty burrs out. I hobbled back inside and put my sandals on.

Without looking up from his book, my dad said, "Never turn your back on Africa."

My mom gave Klaus and me a few days to acclimate to our new world before we had to start school. I was curious to see what we would be learning and how it would differ from a classroom with Mrs. Daniels. I wouldn't be able to get away with as much. No more spitballs or sarcastic comments; it would be too easy for her to tell who did it.

My mom loved animals, and it came across in our studies. My favorite assignment was Insect of the Day. Klaus and I would go find one new insect each day, and most of the time, we didn't have to leave the house. We had a book we searched through to identify it.

At home, in Minnesota, I had my own zoo: fish, birds, countless hamsters, a dog, turtles, and lizards. In Africa, amazing animals were all around us, and our home was part of their unique ecosystem. Geckos came out at night, and we would watch them lick bugs off our ceiling. A wide range of ants were present at all hours of the day, cleaning up after us. They would make thick veins, and I once saw a mass of them carrying a dead gecko up the wall. They were the garbagemen of the world, always picking up debris.

I had lots of "insect time," because the TV sure wasn't like back home. Here, we had four channels, all in languages I did not understand. Every time I turned it on, it was the news. Once I was lucky enough to catch a Bobby McFerrin concert, and I'm still a fan to this day.

When you're home-schooled, it's learning around the clock, not just learning in the time frame of a school day. It's easy to learn about things you're interested in, but math and social studies were like pulling teeth. To me, knowing which bush had the burrs around it was much more useful information. My mother encouraged that approach, and it's something I've carried with me through life: the desire to know more about my surroundings every day.

Other professors and their families lived in the loop of houses, and I was delighted that the family to the right of us had three boys and a daughter near my age. Professor Laleyê and his family were from Benin, another West African country. Klaus and I quickly bonded with the youngest son, Alexander. One morning, he eagerly invited us over and proudly displayed a dead four-foot monitor lizard, riddled with pitchfork holes and dark-red blood oozing out.

"He came in the night and was eating our pigeon and chicken eggs," Alexander explained, poking at it with his toe.

When we told my mom, she said, "Ask if we can have it. We can dissect it and see how it works," which isn't a typical Midwestern mom thing to say. The Lalèyê seemed unsettled by their new White neighbor's odd request.

But they gave it to us.

In the shade of the back porch, we plopped the lizard on its back on a newspaper we couldn't read. Klaus and my mom did the cutting while I did the extraction. We found pieces of eggshells in the guts. I still have the skin to this day. As I write this, I can look up and see the pitchfork holes.

My mom had a book on West African reptiles ready to go, and she made us identify the lizard. We learned it was a savannah monitor; they use their long tail as a whip for primary defense. Later, that information came in handy when Alexander and I chased a six-foot water monitor into an abandoned resort building. Once it was cornered, it turned on us and cracked its bullwhip of a tail, sending us scrambling for home.

The dilapidated resort was a half mile from the university, right on the Senegal River. It was surrounded by a bunch of ramshackle little tourist huts.

"This was going to be a vacation spot for foreigners, but they ran into local opposition and had to abandon the project," Alexander told me. It was heaven for teenage boys who didn't have TV.

Alexander taught me how to fish with a stick, a line, and a hook. We spent the afternoon filling a bucket with banana-sized black catfish and bringing them back to the pond we had dug. It was a concrete basin, 10 feet long, 4 feet wide, and 4 feet deep. It had been intended for some type of water purification but was abandoned, and then it was eventually filled with sand by the relentless Saharan wind. We spent several days digging it out, then dragging the hose from Alexander's yard across the street to fill the pond. Luckily, the school paid for utilities.

We dumped the bucket of catfish into the murky water and never saw them again.

In addition to working with animals, my mom had us pick one African country to do a report on. There were maybe sixty-two to choose from. I forget exactly how many there were at the time, but I chose Nigeria. We also had to learn the names and capitals of all of them. The easiest one to remember—and the most fun to say—was that the capital of Djibouti is Djibouti.

My dad set up an interview for me with one of his Nigerian colleagues who told me his homeland should be one of the wealthiest countries in the world on natural resources alone: diamonds, timber, and oil. But like the rest of Africa, corruption kept it poor.

Another major part of our curriculum was African-American history. We learned in depth about the Civil Rights Movement. We read an amazing book titled *Eyes on the Prize*, where we learned about Emmet Till, Martin Luther King Jr., the Freedom Riders, and Malcom X. My mom read us Maya Angelou's *I Know Why the Caged Bird Sings*, bringing me to tears which I tried to conceal from Klaus. Learning African-American studies in the land of

Africa had so much more of a punch than if I had been sitting in a high school classroom in America, listening to my White teacher regurgitate the same half-truths he had been spouting for the last thirty years. I doubted these books were on the shelves of my school library. And if they were, someone is trying to remove them as I write this. Oh shit, now this book is on the chopping block.

The thing that stuck with me most was our visit to The Door of No Return on the Island of Gorée, just off the coast of Dakar. This was the door which millions of slaves were funneled through before they were forced onto ships bound for the New World. Seeing a photo of that door in a textbook would not have haunted me the way standing in the doorway did. I thought about my African-American friends, about their ancestors being torn from their homes. It made it more real in a way I'll never forget.

My sisters visited and took Klaus and me for a day trip to the beach. We went to the northern border of Senegal, right up against Mauritania. The sand on the beach was extremely hot until you reached the line of sea treasures that were coughed up by the Atlantic. Klaus and I ran ahead of my sisters toward the invisible border of Mauritania; there was no formal crossing, just more sand. It was peaceful. You could see the Sahara pushing down on the ocean and the ocean pushing right back. There were no fishermen on the beach, no goats eating trash, just rolling sand and a couple of coconut trees providing enough shade to the four of us. The waves were massive and dangerous but offset by the gentle sea breeze.

We had a picnic of fruits and sugared peanuts that we bought at the vibrant, chaotic outdoor market en route to the beach. While we ate, my sisters took turns reading aloud from the classic novel *A Separate Peace*. I remember again trying not to cry in front of Klaus. I distracted myself with the big waves, wiping tears as I turned away. After the book was finished, we ran into the water to wash off our sadness while my sisters gathered up our sandy belongings.

The waves scared me. Earlier in the week my dad told us about some students from the university who went to the beach for a field trip. They came back with one less student. He had been sucked into the sea and drowned. I wondered if he had turned his back on the ocean.

We headed back down the shoreline toward civilization, running and playing in the crashing waves. I was looking forward to a bottle of Coke my sisters had promised to buy me back in the market, because my mother didn't let me have sugary drinks. When we got to the invisible border of Senegal, we saw fishermen, children, and animals running on the beach. In the distance there was a man approaching, frantically waving his arms. We figured he was just trying to sell the White people some sort of trinket until he got close enough for his panicked words to reach us: "You're playing in a minefield!"

We froze our frolicking for a second to assess our situation, and then, without discussion, booked it toward him. He told us in a mixture of French and English, "There was a border war ten years ago. It's over, but this is Africa. You never know if they got all the mines."

()()()

On the campus, there were four American exchange students from the University of Madison, Wisconsin, and they treated our house like the American embassy. They would come for my mom's home cooking, escaping the dreaded cafeteria. They brought a welcomed, bright new dynamic to our family. We had the *Saturday Night Live* book *Deep Thoughts* by Jack Handy, and most nights after dinner, the four students would take turns reading from it out loud. We laughed until we pig-snorted.

I have always been a pyromaniac. I love the crackle and pop of fire. I built a fire pit in our yard and spent the days gathering prickly firewood hoping the American students would come entertain me at night. We sat under the stars in the cool sand and talked about home and foods that we missed. I fed the fire until all the fuel was gone.

I was never good at making paper airplanes, my creations would never be approved by the FAA, but one afternoon after class I got the bright idea to light my airborne atrocities on fire. My plan was to send the flaming planes into the meticulously groomed bushes in our front yard, and the fire would burn away the old brown needles that were intertwined with the green needles. My planes were already unpredictable, but it's particularly hard to get a burning paper airplane to land anywhere near where you want it to land. Eventually, I simply just jammed a paper airplane in the bush, and lit it on fire. Gentle reader, I cannot stress enough: Do not do this.

I learned that just because the needles were green didn't mean they weren't as flammable as kerosene. The bush went up like a discarded Christmas tree. Within seconds, the flames were above my head, and I let loose a panicked shriek. The only thing at hand was a cardboard box, and I smacked the fire with it several times, thinking I could smash it out, but this only fanned the flames. I ran to the spigot, but of course the hose was not attached. I tried to fill the cardboard box with water—an exercise in futility. By this time, the flames were roaring 20 feet high.

I fled to the back of the house so I could innocently come running to help and inquire about what had happened once other people took notice. Before I could make my move, the front door banged open, and Klaus rushed out carrying a pot of water. Then came the rest of the bucket brigade: my mom followed by my dad. Everyone's eyes were bulging at the wall of fire.

Before we were able to extinguish the flames, Professor Lalèyê's voice came booming over the fence from the next yard. *"Est-ce que tout va bien là-bas?"*

"Everything's fine!" replied my dad as thick, gray smoke billowed up into the clear blue sky, visible for miles in every direction.

By the time the fire was out, the top half of the bush was gone, and neighbors from all sides came to admire my work. My mom inquired what had happened.

"I wanted to see God?"

Somehow, as miraculous as the burning bush, I never got in trouble and was free to continue my pyromaniacal pursuits. The poor bush never recovered, and every new guest asked why we had three perfectly symmetrical bushes and a charred one. My parents would always refer the guests to me, where I would regale them with the latest version of the tale.

After the paper airplane lesson, my mom redirected my studies to things that flew on their own. She is a bird lover. They were never my favorite of the animal kingdom, but the diversity we had in our own backyard could not be ignored. In addition, 55 kilometers north of us was the Djoudj National Bird Sanctuary, a

UNESCO World Heritage Centre and home to one and a half million boring-ass birds. My highlight of the park was the twenty-foot crocodile, lazily sunning itself on the muddy shore. But the trip to get there was the real adventure.

My parents, Klaus, and I were taking the *car rapide* for a day of study at the park. The car rapide is a bush bus, halfway between a short bus and a regular bus; the outside is painted with vibrant colors of happy faces, religious quotes, and music notes. There was room for ten people, usually jammed with twenty, all entering through the back door. A young man hanging off the back yelled the destination and collected your fare: "Dakar, Dakar, Dakar!"

The luggage and livestock stacked on top doubled the height of the vehicle. You'd get the guy's attention, and he'd tap on the bus with a coin to get the driver to slow down enough for you to jump on.

When we'd stop at an intersection, women would swarm the bus selling bowls of fruit, nuts, and bags of water elegantly teetering on their heads. The food was displayed at the same level as the bus windows. You'd quickly haggle the price, reach out and grab your item, then thrust your money out the window and hopefully get your change before the bus took off again.

The last leg of the journey was an impossible sand road that took forever. The bus never stopped anywhere long enough for me to relieve my bladder, which was fixing to pop. There was nowhere to pee except public spaces; if we exited the bus so I could pee in private, we would have to wait for the next one, which probably wouldn't come until the next day.

The bus got stuck in the sand, wheels spinning uselessly, and my luck turned: something burned out in the engine. Though this gave me the opportunity to pee, there was nary a tree or bush in sight. We were on the edge of the ever-encroaching Sahara Desert.

"Do you know that the United States could fit entirely into the Sahara Desert?" my dad asked, always spouting off trivial encyclopedic information. "That even includes Alaska!"

I scrambled off the bus to find a place to relieve myself.

Way off in the distance, with the distorted heat radiating off the baking sand, I could see a lake of pink. *Is this a mirage?* The pink separated itself from the water, and I realized it was thousands of flamingos taking off at once. This was the border of the Djoudj National Bird Sanctuary, but it was still painfully far away. There was no civilization in sight, but passengers started getting off the bus and trudging down the sand road in random directions. They knew the bus would probably never start again.

Back within the shade of the car rapide, I was telling my mom about the flamingos, when the woman sitting next to me bent down and reached between my legs, underneath my seat. With one hand, she dragged out a hog-tied goat, and then one, two, three white chickens. I had no idea they were even there. Just then, the engine reluctantly started with a cough, and black smoke puffed out of the exhaust.

"*Allah baaxna,*" I said in a combination of Arabic and Wolof, loud enough for everyone to hear. *God is good.*

The six or seven people who remained on the bus cheered at the little toubab's exclamation. The woman next to me began stuffing her livestock back under my seat. Then the engine sputtered out.

"*Allah baaxul,*" I said. *God is bad.*

My dad gasped and clapped his hand over my mouth with a look of terror. He was no doubt personally offended by my blasphemy, but also trying to prevent me from getting stoned or beheaded. Before my offense could register, the engine started up again, and we were on our way to see the boring-ass birds.

For my sixteenth birthday, the four American exchange students took Klaus and me to their favorite bar, Ponky Village. It was a hole-in-the-wall with holes in the walls. There were more mangy dogs and cats than patrons. We sat on the patio, enclosed with bougainvillea bushes. The bar was nestled at the quiet end of Saint Louis Island, and thirty yards from the bar, the mighty Senegal River at its widest and most polluted pushed by toward the Atlantic. I saw a sheep, up to its filthy fleece in the dirty water, eating wet trash.

At the table, I ordered my first of one million beers in a bar. The brand was called Gazelle. I don't know how many ounces it was, but the bottle was bigger than my head. I was feeling pretty good by the time we ordered. The students raved about the *poulet yassa*, which is onions and chicken on top of white rice.

I stumbled half-drunk, half-palsy to the bathroom. When I turned on the light, the walls and floor crawled to life with a carpet of roaches. The toilet was a slippery hole in the ground that had never been cleaned. I wished I had my trusty billy club, although this was really more of a job for a flamethrower. I peed in the general direction of the hole from the doorway and all but ran back to my seat.

When I returned to the table, as is always the case, the food had arrived, although I had left my appetite back in the bathroom. I ordered another beer instead of eating and wondered what my parents would think if they knew the students were letting us drink. The tantalizing aroma of the poulet yassa won me over, and I eagerly wolfed it down before ordering another beer for the road.

By this time I was quite drunk, and there was some concern I would fall into the river. We were heading to another bar, but I insisted we first stop at a gelato stand. The Senegalese woman behind the counter was the most beautiful I had ever seen; very tall, with even taller cheekbones. I wanted there to be an ice cream flavor as rich and dark as her skin. Liquid courage got my French and Wolof flowing smoothly. She laughed and smiled and flirted back.

"What's your name?" she asked, handing me a chocolate gelato.

"My name is Babakar," I replied in Wolof.

With that, her smile disappeared, and she looked into my soul as she grabbed my good arm. "No. From now on, you will be called Bamba."

Whatever you say, pretty lady. I melted away to let the other people order.

I sat on a high curb to eat my dripping dessert in a spot where I could wait for my friends and still watch her scoop gelato. A tall, stunningly handsome man with perfect dreadlocks awkwardly sat next to me, his knees up around his shoulders like a giant grasshopper. At this point in the night I was feeling more than good. I had beer, sugar, and electric energy from flirting coursing through me. The man mirrored my mood.

"Your Wolof is better than most toubab," he said. "What do they call you?"

"Bamba," I said, gazing back at the beauty behind the counter.

"That is a very powerful name you have. Sheikh Ahmadou Bamba is one the greatest spiritual leaders of Senegal. He fought colonialism."

"I didn't know all that," I said, "she just gave me the name."

"Ah, yes, she is very beautiful."

"I want her to be my wife," I said in Wolof.

"Yes," he laughed as he reached down and patted my dick. "What are you going to do with that?"

I was drunk enough to laugh and make a lewd gesture, which I am pretty sure Sheikh Ahmadou Bamba would not approve of.

From that point on, my name in Senegal was Bamba. I had accepted it out of teen horniness, but it stuck, and I still use it to this day.

◯◯◯

My dad was a smoker for the longest time, but he pretended none of us knew. He used to go out for walks and come back smelling like Life Savers and cheap African cigarettes. After one of those walks, he burst through the door, panicked and winded: "Those feral dogs started following me. I had to throw rocks to keep them away." He checked the window to see if they were gathering in the yard.

While I thought it was funny and just an overreaction at the time, I would soon have my own run-in with the pack.

After my daily explorations, I would often head back outside to stare at the stars. There were different constellations here than in the cold Minnesota skies. Some nights I ventured beyond the well-lit safety of our fenced yard. When the streetlights went out along the barely paved roads, the stars would shine brighter. The streetlights along the professor's loop were like slow flashing Christmas lights, as if there was only enough electricity to light up a handful of bulbs at a time. Sometimes a patch of three streetlights would go out in a row, and I would get a brilliant view of the sky. When the lights came back on, I'd move around the circle, chasing after the pools of darkness.

I was gazing up at the sky one night, and the light directly above me clicked on. I blinked, looked away, and on the outer edge of the light circle was one of those feral dogs lazily loping behind me. The light abruptly clicked off, giving me back the stars but leaving me to wonder what the dog was up to. I closed my eyes to readjust them to the darkness. When I opened them, the dog had moved considerably closer, and it now had a dirty companion. A couple of streetlights ahead, the light came on. Now there were three dogs.

I fought back the urge to shriek and run to the safety of the next streetlight, as if it were base, and somehow, the dogs knew the rules of the game. I knew that would give the dogs more incentive to chase, and as soon as I got there, it would probably click back off, anyway. I kept my same pace, and in the time it would have taken me to run there, the light did go out. All the hair on my neck went up, and I snarled. My body tensed, and it wasn't the palsy. I was being hunted. I was now halfway around the circle, still moving but definitely no longer paying attention to the stars.

Usually, I carried at least one weapon, like the roach-killing billy club, or my homemade bow and arrow, but that night, I didn't even have my slingshot. In what little light I had, I scanned the ground. It was all sand. Where had my dad found rocks to throw at them?

A light blinked. Now all the dogs were there. I didn't know how many, but I knew it was the full pack. As I rounded the bend, I could see the safety of our porch light and our fenced yard. The street lights went out again. The dogs were painfully silent. I kept moving toward home, and by the time I got to our front gate, I was alone again. My mangy, worm-bitten stalkers had left me at the edge of the light. They knew I had made it to safety.

From that point on I always traveled around the neighborhood with my wrist rocket slingshot and a pocketful of pebble projectiles.

Whenever I ventured outside in the hottest part of the day, my mom would sing a line from an old show tune: "Only mad dogs and Englishmen go out in the midday sun."

I would laugh as I ran out into the hot world; there were too many things to explore, and a day without a middle wasn't long enough for me. Plus it was nice to get away from the singing.

Once outside my fence I saw the pack. They were dozing in the shade of the acacia trees at the center of the housing loop. We had been in a stalemate ever since a few days prior when I fired rocks at them with my slingshot to show them I was not to be trifled with.

But I couldn't let sleeping dogs lie.

The day was especially hot; even their usual sentry had dozed off. Guided by primal instinct and supreme stupidity, I crept toward my pet project, slingshot at the ready. When none of them awoke, I decided to see how far into the slumbering pack I could get. There were thirteen dogs spread out so they had space to sleep without touching. I found a thorn-free spot at the edge, palsy-picked my way to the middle of the pack, and sat down.

A fly left one of the dogs to come explore me. It landed on my arm and sucked up a bead of sweat. The dogs were skinny and mangy, with open sores. Bits of their ears had been eaten away by flies, and gunk crusted with sand trailed down from their eyes like painful tears.

I must have sat there for almost ten minutes before one dog at the edge of the pack lazily picked its head up, saw me, and did a double-take. It's the only animal I've ever seen do a double-take. It jumped up and made one low call, letting the others know there was something weird going on. With that the rest of the dogs jumped up. Now all eyes were fixed on me with a look of confused canine embarrassment. A few nights ago I had been potential prey, and now, I had infiltrated their comfort zone, surprising them in a way that no human had before.

One by one they slunk away. After that, the pack gave me a wide berth, unsure what to make of this strange primate, although I often felt them watching me as I explored the bush. I had earned their begrudging respect.

Sometimes stupidity pays off.

I spent a lot of time with the Laléyê family next door. We communicated in a mixture of French and English and would try out our Wolof on each other. While I had first connected with Alexander, over time the middle son Xavier became my best friend. Xavier would smile and say to me in French: "You are my brother, but you fell into the flour," to which I would reply, "and you are my brother, but you fell into the charcoal."

Xavier and I loved playing soccer. He was a great goalie. I had an enviable soccer ball I brought from the States, and he would let me take shots at him. I think I only scored five times over the course of a year, but in my defense he was quite a bit taller than I was.

And didn't have palsy.

The layout of our homes was almost identical, except for the full-blown farm they had in their yard, including pigeons, rabbits, chickens, and a friendly goat. All of this was very alluring. Like my mother, I love animals. I would hang out with their menagerie while the kids were at school. The sweet, funny goat was my favorite.

Madame Lalèyê had a regal presence that reminded me of Mrs. Daniels. Her personality matched the vibrant colors that she wore, and she was a hell of a cook. If soccer was the universal language between Xavier and me, cooking was the language of our mothers. Despite speaking different languages, they would come together and swap recipes and techniques.

But I'll most remember Madame Lalèyê for saving me from a terrible illness.

I had a high fever, diarrhea, and projectile vomiting for two delirious weeks. I was unable to even keep water down. My parents took me to a doctor who prescribed western medicine that had no effect on my symptoms. My mom was concerned, because I was losing weight. Madame Lalèyê showed up on our doorstep with a big mason jar full of a grayish liquid with sticks and leaves floating in it. She produced a shot glass out of the wrinkles in her flowered robe and filled it with the mysterious liquid. She explained to my parents in French that I needed to gargle the concoction for one minute.

They brought the slimy, gray liquid to my bed, which had been moved to the living room so that I could be social while I died. I did as instructed and spat the disgusting bitter contents into a bowl. My dad, sitting blithely nearby on the couch doing a crossword puzzle, looked up. "Josh, did you know the word for tree in Wolof is the same as the word for medicine?"

The next morning, the effects were nothing short of a miracle.

My fever had dropped, and I felt like I was stumbling out of a foggy tunnel. I had my first real drink of water in days.

When Xavier wasn't in school, and I wasn't actively dying of a mysterious waterborne illness, we spent our free time running through the bush, throwing rocks and shooting slingshots at each other. We would usually round out our day with two games of chess. We were evenly matched and would win one each, but neither one of us had the attention span for the tiebreaker.

Our favorite game was playing war with broomstick guns; hunting each other through the four-story abandoned dorms the university had been building until they ran out of funds. These unforgiving concrete shells had no glass in the windows or roofs overhead, and a good two inches of dust on the floor. Every time we visited, there were new, perfect animal tracks, but the only human footprints were ours from previous battles. Huge barn owls roosted on the top floors of every dorm, nine of them, which Xavier avoided at all costs. He warned me to do the same and explained that owls are Africa's Grim Reaper.

I was coming to find an Africa full of mysteries that challenged my western beliefs. Xavier told me when he was a kid in Benin, he had a high fever for several days. On the third night an owl flew into his room. In many African cultures, the owl is a harbinger of death, helping guide souls to the next world. The owl flew in frantic circles over Xavier's bed, and his father rushed in with a broom, swatting the bird until it flew back out. The next day Xavier felt one hundred percent better.

But where I come from, owls are cool. So I would regularly visit them by myself, sneaking up to the top floors of the abandoned dorms to hang out with them. Despite how quietly I moved, every time I peeked around the corner, the owl was already staring deep into my soul with its luminous golden eyes. After an unsettling staring contest, which I always won, the owl would turn and fly out the window. Beneath its perch was a mound of pellets two feet high. I'd scoop them up, ten at a time, to add to my mom's unique curriculum. We'd dissect them and might find six different animals in one pellet, from small rodents to large, long-legged birds.

One evening, during a chess game in the Lalèyê's front yard, with my goat buddy bleating in the background, I told Xavier how much I hated going to church. "I don't believe in God," I said.

Eyes wide, Xavier asked, "How can you not believe in God?"

"I don't believe in someone who would put me on Earth in this broken body," I said, gesturing to my right arm.

"Maybe you just don't see how lucky you are," he replied. "If you were born here, you'd be dead by now."

"I *was* born here," I reminded him. He responded with a look that told me to shut the fuck up. But I knew what he meant. I was fortunate enough to be medevaced out of Cameroon shortly after my birth. If I hadn't been born to a rich *toubab* family with the ability to get to a good hospital, I would have been visited by an owl. Living in Africa helped me realize that just because I have a physical disability doesn't mean I don't have a lot of other spectacular things in my life.

Things like food, shelter, water. You know, the little things.

Often after our games of chess, Xavier invited me to stay for lunch. I never turned down Madame Lalèyê's outstanding cooking. As delicious as the food was, I learned a painful lesson in asking for specifics about what was on the menu.

One afternoon, after another outstanding meal, I went outside to visit the animals. When I got to the goat's pen, it was ominously empty. My full stomach dropped as I ran back to the kitchen. *"Où est mon ami?"* I shouted.

Xavier gave me a smirk and raised his eyebrow at my belly. "You know where your friend is!"

The oldest Lalèyê brother bent down and opened the oven door, revealing my friend's head on a cookie sheet. "It's the best part," he said in French, poking at the charred cheek.

And worst of all, that was not the last friend I ate.

A few days later, Klaus found a white puppy on his afternoon jog. Much to the chagrin of my father, my mom said we could keep it. I was overjoyed and came up with the perfect name for him: Toubab! We soon learned it was a terrible idea to invite a feral animal into your home. Toubab was a terror and resisted learning even the simplest of commands.

He was voracious but had little use for chewing his food and chewed everything else indiscriminately. As soon as you turned your back, he was on the table in a flash and could eat a baguette in two bites. He harassed our chickens and used our house like a toilet. He was an all around pain in the ass. Throughout the day, we yelled at the dog endlessly. My dad pointed out that our Wolof-speaking neighbors must think we are insane. It did sound like White people scolding each other:

"Toubab! Drop it!"

"Toubab bit me!"

"Toubab shat on my bed again!"

A month later, our gardener showed up with another white puppy, thinking the silly toubabs were running a shelter. Much to the joy of my father, my mom said, "One is more than enough, but the Lalèyês don't have a dog. Why don't you put it in their yard?"

And so that's what he did.

The next day, before morning lesson, I went across the street to check on the fish pond, and there was the puppy, floating belly up in the murky water. After the initial shock, I went to the house to get Klaus and a shovel. As we buried the puppy, we discussed not telling my parents. I didn't want my mom to feel responsible.

A week later, my dad came to the breakfast table, looking rather peaked. "I know this sounds crazy, but every night for the last week when I get up to go to the bathroom, out of the corner of my eye I see a small white dog in the hallway. When I turn the flashlight toward it, it's not there. I thought maybe Toubab had escaped, but I check every time, and he's always locked in the kitchen, asleep."

Across the table, Klaus' wide-eyed face mirrored my own. I spoke first. "So, you guys remember that puppy?" I looked to Klaus for reassurance. "The Lalèyês didn't keep it. Alexander told me they wanted a male dog, so they let it out of their yard. I guess it must have been thirsty and went to drink from our fish pond and fell in and drowned. Klaus and I buried it."

My dad sat there slack-jawed. "Where did you bury it?"

Klaus spoke up. "We buried it in the sand, right next to the pond."

My dad turned toward my mom; she was sad but stoic. He now looked ghostly and fragile and slowly pushed himself away from the table. "Please don't tell anyone. My colleagues will frown upon the White people summoning ghosts."

He walked away, leaving a collective *what the fuck* hanging over the table.

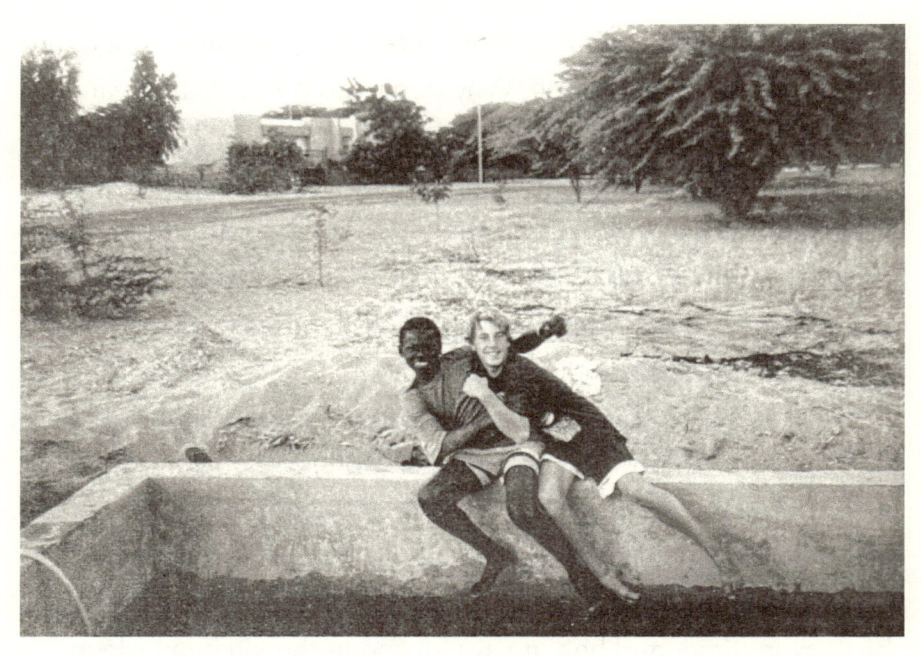

Me and Alexander wrestling by the pond we dug inside the professors' housing loop.

That night, Klaus and I were terrified of the ghost puppy's revenge, yet kind of hoping to see her again. The next morning my dad sat down like it wasn't on all of our minds.

"Well, did you see it?" I asked.

"No," he said with an air of relief.

I was a bit disappointed.

"Maybe the dog just wanted to be recognized," my dad said.

He was right, because the dog never returned in our time there. But I like to think that she did return to terrify every other exchange professor who dared to stay there.

()()()

After living in Africa for almost a year, we returned home to Minnesota. I was surprised to have more culture shock coming back than when I left. I would turn on the water and think, *you mean I can just drink this, raw?* And I could sleep at night knowing my home was free of ghost puppies. The pace of everything was fevered in the States. Rush, rush, rush, everyone was in a hurry to get nowhere. If Africa time meant you were two hours late, America time meant it should have happened yesterday.

It was the summer after Senegal, I was 16 years old, and my parents weren't sure what to do with me. They enrolled me in a summer work program for inner city youth. The program had us doing "easy" construction jobs that weren't worth bringing in a real crew: building cinder-block walls, putting up heavy guardrails on the freeway, and digging. So much digging. We were a chain gang without chains. It was a group of Somali, Latino, Vietnamese, and Hmong boys, with a disabled *toubab* in the mix.

I remember one kid would rather sit in the porta-potty than work. He'd say, "I really gotta go," while bouncing on one foot, and then be in there for hours over the course of the day until the laid-back director would come and pound on the porta-potty door and coax him out with an offer of lunch or a legit break. He would emerge glistening from the humidity of the baking hot plastic shit box, eager to eat.

It was a seven-week program that ate up my whole summer. Every couple weeks I got a small paycheck, which I spent on fast food, thrift store jeans, grunge CDs, and candy.

The director loved me. I entertained him by talking trash about my peers, forming a bond. At the end of the program he took me to a Neil Young concert, teaching me the valuable lesson: being a smart-ass can pay off.

A recruiter came and told us we were invited to substitute a week of work in the city for a week at a wilderness work camp called Camp Sunrise in Rush City, Minnesota. We were taking the chain gang on the road. After my mom eagerly signed the permission slip for me to go away for a week, they added that this was where *The Children of the Corn* was filmed.

Before I knew it, I was off on a school bus heading north with thirty boys I did not know. I could tell most of them had never seen more than two trees next to each other; this was going to be their first camp experience.

As the bus worked its way down the dusty dirt road into camp, I could see in the distance a diverse group of people playing volleyball, most of them wearing red or blue bandanas, which I immediately related to Crips and Bloods. I started worrying that my parents got me caught up in some sort of gang camp.

We pulled to a stop. I saw the mass of campers and realized I was going to be one of the only White people, and definitely the only physically disabled person at sunny Camp Sunrise. The palms of my hands started sweating. I hadn't been on such an adventure since Senegal.

A large face with an eye patch and a blue bandana looked into my soul through the school bus window with his one, dazzling eye. "Welcome to camp," he said in an accented, low tone.

He scared the shit out of me. I later found out that the one eye belonged to a Zairian counselor named Samson, and I definitely knew I did not want him as my counselor.

The campers were broken down into A, B, C, and D crews. You were expected to instantly develop a blinding loyalty to your crew. Which I still do to this day…B Crew for life! There were eight boys to a crew between the ages of 12 and 17, a head counselor, an assistant counselor, and if you were lucky, a cute junior counselor. Our crew was only seven strong, but we were a lot to handle for our college-aged counselors.

Our head counselor was a tall, skinny Black woman named Tanya who never removed her blue bandana. The assistant counselor was Janice, a short Black woman who never removed her red bandana.

Name games (which induced more hand sweating due to the fear of my own voice), snacks, and a breakdown of what the week would look like ensued. The event that loomed large in my mind was the skit we were required to perform at the end of the week. Fortunately, there were enough other fun, terrifying activities to distract me.

The first night was easy. They had four boys to each platform canvas tent, and I was in the tent of three. After dinner it was slapping mosquitoes and playing basketball on the uneven dirt court. The beat-up hoop was nailed to a tree trunk and abnormally high. I suck at basketball; I can run and kick all day, but dribbling with my hands is not in my skill set. I was entranced by the bouncing ball. Every time it hit the ground, a poof of dust flew up.

Somewhere in the mix, two boys butted heads. Shouts between them turned into shoving. As it escalated, I watched Samson approach the boys with calm, long strides. Right before it came to blows, he stepped between them and said in his deep baritone, "Real men fight naked."

And with that, the fight was over. The boys went back to playing basketball, but they were clearly off their game, still processing Samson's thought-provoking wisdom.

Camp Sunrise was on the Minnesota side of the pristine St. Croix River. During the week, we were to take a three-day canoe trip down the river, camping and cleaning the shores, as we paddled our way back to Camp Sunrise from the drop-off point upstream. At the end of the trip, the collected trash would be weighed, and the winners would get first dibs on the barbecued chicken dinner when we returned.

There were several launch points to choose from, and B Crew picked the farthest one, to the dismay of our counselors.

"That's very ambitious," Tanya said with an air of dread, cutting a glance at Janice. "We will be paddling more than playing, just so you know."

Our eager boy imaginations persisted with the 56-mile paddle despite the fact that none of us had ever canoed before. Once on the water, we discovered we were ill-equipped to travel six miles, let alone fifty-six. I quickly had to learn my own unique paddling style, as I could only paddle on the left side of the boat but needed to be able to steer in both directions. The counselors may have originally thought that the disabled kid would need the most help, but as the canoe trip wore on, they came to realize I was more than capable of keeping up physically and also able to assist others by helping set up tents, etc.

B Crew consisted of quite a cast of characters. The hefty cornerstone was a boy named Gerard, two years younger, but twice my size. Always complaining about his swollen ankles and his inability to eat cheese, he sounded more like an aged Southern belle than an inner-city boy from the streets of Minneapolis.

"Too much cheddar cheese blocks me up," he would say as he rubbed his round belly. He was less than capable of paddling a canoe full of camping gear.

On the first day he was my canoe partner. It was like riding a teeter-totter. His end rode very low, and on my end I could barely reach the water with my paddle. Eventually, Tanya moved all the gear toward me as a counterweight so that the wind stopped spinning us around like a top.

On the second day the counselors realized Gerard would be better off treated like luggage and sat him on the bottom of the canoe, in the middle, between myself and another unlucky camper. We paddled him down the river like an Egyptian goddess as he complained and mowed through our snacks.

Anytime we complained about our sunburns, mosquito bites, or blistered palms, Tanya and Janice reminded us through gritted teeth that *we* chose this distance despite their warnings. Later I overheard Tanya bitching to Janice in their tent, "I'm never giving kids the choice of fifty-six miles again."

The real troublemaker of B Crew was a tall, slender kid with an afro and a missing front tooth, who didn't participate in anything. I mentally gave him the very clever nickname Missing Tooth.

Missing Tooth would shout, "Why does the fat kid get to ride in the sweet spot?"

I could see Janice resist the urge to yell back, "Because he's the fucking fat kid!"

We limped back to Camp Sunrise hours past our expected arrival, and the barbecue had already started. I was sunburnt and haggard from the journey, but over the past three days I had fallen in love with the river and canoeing, while my crewmates were ready to retreat back home to the city.

At dinner, I was eager to get away from the drama of B Crew so I went to see what other crews had to offer. I sat with a couple of boys from D Crew and talked shit about the troublemakers from my trip. I pointed out Swollen Ankles gnawing on a block of forbidden cheddar cheese.

The kids in D Crew told me that on their canoe trip, Samson took off his eye patch and popped in a thousand-dollar glass eye. They said they were splashing around in the shallow beach area, and Samson's eye fell out into the river. Thrashing furiously up and down the shore, he screamed "Help me find my eye!" He had all eight boys in D Crew knee-deep in the river, combing the water for three hours. The kids said a fat Wisconsin fisherman had floated by, slack-jawed at the unlikely scene before him.

I looked over at Samson at the next table. He had his eye patch back on and the body posture of a man who had lost his thousand-dollar eye. "So you're telling me there's a thousand-dollar eye still out there?" I asked, imagining a family picnic ruined by that gruesome discovery.

Toward the end of the week, I was moseying along the trail without any real purpose, when Stephanie, the assistant director of the camp, walked by me. "How's it going?" she said with a smile as we passed each other.

"Splendid."

She laughed at my genuine response. "You're always in such a great mood. You fit in great here."

My smile broadened. *I fit in somewhere?*

In keeping with tradition, the whole camp gathered around the bonfire to pass the sacred canoe paddle and give a brief summary of what they would take away from their Camp Sunrise experience. The paddle had been in the hand of every camper and counselor at Camp Sunrise for twenty-five years.

But first we had to survive the skits I was dreading all week. The first skit was with my crew. We tried to re-enact some of the choice moments from our canoe trip, although these were inside jokes only B Crew got. Most of the kids were better at canoeing than acting, except for Swollen Ankles who had a pleasantly commanding stage presence.

I shined in my second skit where Stephanie and I did impressions of "Klaus & Franz," the bodybuilders from *Saturday Night Live*. We stuffed our sweatpants full of pillows and put sweatshirts over life jackets so we had big barrel chests.

"I am Klaus, and this is Franz, and we are here to pump—*clap*—you up." Our timing on the clap was perfect.

Looking back, I recognize that doing *SNL* impressions isn't the height of comedy, but this was my first taste of performing and we got big laughs from my target audience, the counselors.

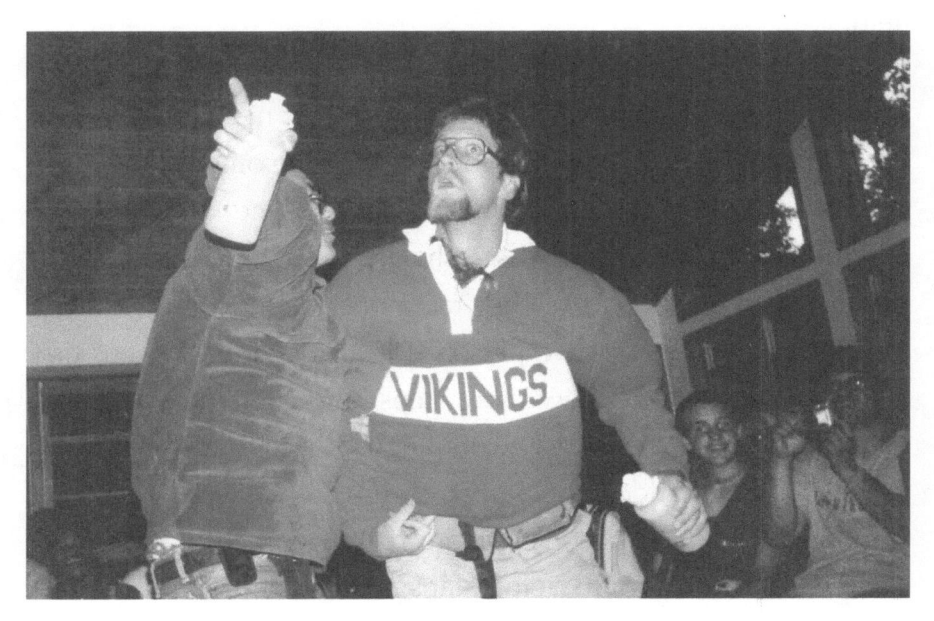

I'm here to pump you up.

My nervousness was still there, but once I got onstage, everything was about being present in the moment. I forgot about my disability and all other concerns. I just made people laugh. I learned much later that comedy also makes the audience present: When you are laughing with everybody else, you're not thinking about your own shitty life.

Shortly after camp ended, I gave the performance of my lifetime. Since Stephanie and I had bonded as Klaus and Franz, I all but begged her and the camp director Flannery to come to my house to teach me how to ride a bike. To my surprise, they agreed.

When they arrived, I met them with my sister's beat-up 10-speed, and we walked to the nearby school. I beamed proudly as I entertained them, enjoying the attention of these older, beautiful women in front of the neighbor kids. We decided not to start off on the asphalt to save me some skin, so we went on the football field.

"Okay, are you ready, Josh?" Flannery asked as she held one side of the bike, which was just a bit too tall for me.

"You got this," Stephanie said, steadying the other side.

They both had a hand on the back of the bike seat and another on the handlebars as I shakily brought my feet to the pedals and started to crank. They ran alongside me for a few steps. Realizing it wasn't a two-person job, Stephanie let go first. Flannery held on for a few more steps, and I whimpered a little when she let go. Then I was wobbling off to the races. I made a big, wide, right-handed circle back toward them.

"You're doing it!" they shouted. "Keep pedaling!"

I took a few more victory laps and guided the bike back between them. I jumped off with a gigantic smile. A glance bounced between the two ladies, the final puzzle pieces coming together.

Stephanie asked, "So Josh, did you know how to ride a bike before we came here?"

I giggled as I rode away into the sunset.

I needed a job the summer after my freshman year in college, and I knew where I wanted to work: sunny Camp Sunrise. Ever since my first visit at sixteen, I loved the camp, and they loved me back. I applied to be a counselor, but they hired me as an assistant counselor, because I don't drive.

School got out late, so I showed up two days before the campers and missed most of the orientation, which was fine by me. My attention span was only good for the length of two chess games, anyway.

Now it was my turn to scare the campers. At the welcome orientation, we all gathered at the central fire pit and went around the circle introducing ourselves. When it was my turn, I bolted up like a tweaker and in a raspy voice said, "I'm Chopsaw, the sworn leader of B Crew."

The counselors laughed. The campers did not. It was clear from their body language that they wanted nothing to do with Chopsaw's crew. The crews were formed, and the unlucky eight reluctantly trudged over to Chopsaw for their sweaty high five, still trying to figure out what my major malfunction was.

I dropped the Chopsaw voice and helped lead the name games, but even so, I rarely knew my campers' names on any given week. I resorted to "dude" and on-the-fly nicknames. I'd see a kid with a big ol' head: "Hey, Pumpkin Patch." Verbal bullying came naturally to me.

When it came to planning the three-day canoe trip, I knew to never offer the 56-mile option. As we stood at the edge of the St. Croix River, ready to embark, I again reminded them that as we were seemingly looking for trash to collect, we were really looking for that thousand-dollar eye (for my own personal collection).

A camper pointed her paddle at me and pleaded to the head counselor, "You want me to get in a boat with *that* man?"

"You are damn lucky to have him on board," the head counselor said.

The campers soon learned that Chopsaw was not only funny but also a reliable source on the river: from putting up tents and building fires to cooking and hanging up food to keep away from pesky bears and raccoons, I could do it all—except drive. They also learned that I was their only way home; we were truly in the wilderness. This was before cell phones. I was their map, GPS, and entertainment. I taught them that nature was beautiful, but emphasized it could also be deadly. I used their ignorance against them. When they resisted bedtime, I told them that the wolves would be out hunting soon, and their giggles sounded a lot like a wounded fawn.

Not only would I get the campers back safely, we would often eat first at the barbecue dinner for collecting the most trash on the river. But perhaps most importantly, at the end of the week, I made sure B Crew's skits were the funniest.

The second summer, they still hadn't promoted me because I still couldn't drive. I was okay with it since it was slightly less responsibility, and it meant I was occasionally paired with Linda, a head counselor and my best friend at camp. We both really enjoyed playing practical jokes on each other. One time, she bored a hole in a brownie with a chopstick, crammed a Thai hot pepper in it, and plugged it back up. She had never given me anything before, except a shitty haircut. I didn't fall for it.

Week four, my dream came true. I was Linda's assistant counselor. Our junior counselor was Bao. We were in charge of the B Crew boys. Linda and Bao were Hmong, and I was absorbing their language without realizing it, just as I had done with Wolof.

Our crew consisted of four Somali boys, three Hmong boys, and Uncle Fester, a bald, pudgy, White boy—I told you I was good with nicknames—with the intelligence of bread dough. Looking back, I realize Uncle Fester was probably on the spectrum, but it was the '90s, and I had no frame of reference for this. But Asperger's was the least of his worries. We were all in the van, and the Somali boys were speaking Arabic. Uncle Fester told me, "Tell them to stop speaking that language."

I said, "Why don't you ask them what language it is and try to learn a few words?"

"Tell them to stop speaking that language," he said again.

No matter what positive solution I pitched, he would always respond with his own special brand of ignorance.

Uncle Fester was especially useless on the canoe trip, more so than Swollen Ankles. After two days on the river, he still did not understand how to paddle, so Linda decided it would be easier to dump him with me while she took on the remaining seven campers. Yeah, easier, for *her*. I sat in the back of the canoe frantically barking orders as we pinballed off rocks, plunging through the rapids.

The other campers hated Uncle Fester. He argued and complained incessantly. You couldn't even play games with the dude. At lunch, while we were all enduring one of his emotional outbursts, a look spread across Linda's face. It was a look of *oh shit!* that transformed to *ohhhh. Shit.* She pulled a ziplock bag from the first-aid kit. "You forgot to tell me to give him his medication!"

"You're the Head Counselor!" I shot back.

Linda fished the medication out of the waterproof bag, and I fed them to Uncle Fester, hoping for some immediate improvement.

Back on the river, I waited for a change, but it never came. At least not in the form of paddling or stopping racist outbursts. Eventually, I told the dude to just quit paddling and sit still so we wouldn't capsize.

By the time we rode ashore to our last campsite, my arms were rubber from a second day of paddling Uncle Fester's dead weight. As you may imagine, gentle reader, I'm a bit dominant on the left side, so I had to both propel and steer the boat from one side. I used what was left of my strength to stabilize the canoe as Uncle Fester wobbled out, walked right to the picnic table, and sat down. He looked waterlogged, even though he was dry.

We set up the camp and prepared dinner while Uncle Fester supervised us. There were three tents, two for the campers and one for the counselors. We were exhausted and needed the boys to go to bed early, so I told them the wolves would be out hunting soon. The three Hmong kids knew there weren't any wolves but shared their tent begrudgingly with Uncle Fester. As Linda, Bao, and I tidied up the campsite, the boys in Tent 2 bickered in Hmong about their tentmate. They only switched to English to berate him.

"You're not supposed to eat in the tent!"

"You're on my side!"

"Oh God, what's that smell?"

After shushing them several times, we finally crawled into our tent, physically and mentally drained.

"What a week!" I said as I zipped up my sleeping bag. I never knew hard ground could feel so good.

"Well, that's the great thing about Camp Sunrise," Linda said. "It will prepare you for anything."

And with that, the brightest flash of electric blue lit up the world, accompanied by a teeth-rattling *boom*. A bolt of lightning struck a nearby tree. Everyone's screams were quickly drowned out by what sounded like a lake being dumped on us. The lightning was so frequent we couldn't tell one blue explosion from another.

Linda unzipped our tent flap. We poked our heads out to find Tent 2 collapsed in on itself. Through the lightning flashes, I could see it was raining so hard there were already pools of water on top of the wriggling tent.

I turned to Linda, expecting her to jump into head counselor action.

"You go!" she said.

"Me?"

Bao nodded in approval.

I took off my dry shirt and plunged into the deluge. My bare feet sank ankle-deep into cold water. For a brief second, my frizzy hair blew in the wind before being drenched and plastered to my head. As I floundered with the wet tent full of scared boys, I could hear them swearing in Hmong. I got hold of the writhing zipper and struggled to open it. Thankfully, the boys were unharmed, at least physically.

"What happened?" I shouted over the rain and thunder.

They all pointed their flashlights at Uncle Fester. I wondered how he could possibly knock a tent down from the inside. But I skipped the question and made a head counselor's decision. "You three sleep in Tent 1," I told the Hmong boys. Then I had Uncle Fester grab his gear to sleep in the counselor's tent.

He slowly and luxuriously gathered his things, emerging into the raging storm in no particular hurry. He slogged his way through the muddy water, dragging his sleeping bag behind him. By the time I got the three boys settled and waded my way back to my tent, Uncle Fester had set up in his soggy sleeping bag—in my spot.

The tent was on a slight incline, and it was conveniently decided while I was out saving everyone, that I would sleep at the low end where the puddle formed. I climbed in over everybody and squeezed beside Uncle Fester. He was soon snoring his heavy fester-breath in my face, drowning out the storm as it rumbled away.

Somewhere in the wee hours, Uncle Fester pissed my sleeping bag. The odor was thick in the humid, confined tent, and the smell permeated my dreams, waking me with wet dread. I realized the situation, but I was so exhausted, there was nothing to do but force myself back to sleep.

I was up with the sun. I ran straight to the river and dove in, half hoping to drown. We had survived the trip, and I somehow resisted the urge to leave Uncle Fester behind in the wilderness for the wolves to clean up.

The next summer, I convinced Liz, my friend from college, to work as a counselor with me. Late in the season, we were paired together to lead the D Crew girls' canoe trip. D Crew for life! In general, girls' weeks were much easier than the testosterone-fueled boys' weeks, so I wasn't dreading the trip. While boys fought over how many raisins were in their granola bar, girls were helpful and actually engaged with the activities.

The first day on the river, we were paddling into our campsite, and a girl nicknamed T started a splash fight. We all got soaked, but she deservedly got the worst of it. While we felt bad for her, it was a hot sunny day, and there was plenty of daylight to spare. T left her drenched jogging suit on as she helped unpack and set up camp; we assumed it would dry quickly.

We ate dinner, the sun set, and it finally cooled down. Liz and I didn't give any thought to T and her wet clothes, it just wasn't that cold. As we all sat around making s'mores and joking around, we realized T was no longer making any sense. Her words were gibberish. Looking closer, she was shivering uncontrollably. I put my shaky hand on her shoulder to steady her and discovered her shirt was still wet, and now cold. We told her she needed to get out of her wet clothes immediately, but she just sat there, unresponsive. T was the loudmouth of the group, so her silence frightened us.

We told the other campers to take T to her tent and get her into dry clothes. Seven concerned girls gently steered her away—like she was an elderly dementia patient who had wandered off. Liz rummaged through the first-aid kit for the small book of ailments. With growing dread, we read the entry for hypothermia by flashlight.

Incoherency: *Check.*
Shivering: *Check.*
Unresponsive: *Check.*

We continued down the list of symptoms until we read—out loud and in unison—the final outcome: Death.

We stared wide-eyed at each other for a moment and then snapped into action. Liz read aloud, "Somebody needs to get into a sleeping bag naked with her."

"Okay *you* do that, I'm running for help."

I had no idea where to go; we were in the middle of nowhere Wisconsin. The moon and stars were bright enough to light a path into the woods, and the trees were shadows cut into the night sky.

Liz had insisted that I bring the most responsible camper with me as backup, and the girl reluctantly came along. I ran as fast as the forest allowed while making sure not to lose the girl following me. As I ran, I had one focus: getting help for T. There was no thought of second-guessing myself based on palsy. After about fifteen minutes of panicked sprinting, the path led to the butt end of a dirt road, and the sky opened up above us. Progress! My winded shadow and I hurried onward.

We ran twenty minutes down the dirt road until we reached a paved T-junction. Then I saw it: a square of light in the distant woods. We fought our way through the brush and discovered a small cabin. I pounded on the door. After a moment a scared old man in his tighty-whities cautiously opened. I was almost too out of breath to speak. "We're having a medical emergency down at the river."

As he assessed us, the look on his face grew more concerned. If they had sent this pair for help—a gasping, wild-eyed monster and an Asian tween—the situation must truly be dire. He led me to his landline; I tried to call 911, but was so shaky I couldn't turn the dial on the ancient green rotary phone. The old-timer stepped in and dialed for me, then handed the phone back.

An ambulance met us at the T-junction a painful thirty minutes later. We got in and led them to our campsite. T was alive, but her teeth were still chattering. The paramedics wrapped her up in a tinfoil blanket like a burrito and loaded her onto a stretcher. Liz went to the hospital with T to look after her and fill out her paperwork—my skill set was better suited for the woods.

At around 3 a.m., Liz crawled back into the tent, exhausted. "The camp wants us to pick up T downriver tomorrow," she said.

This sounded unlikely to me, as T had been near death and was currently in the hospital. But to my surprise, the next day, as we paddled toward a bridge, there was a Camp Sunrise van waiting, with T and the camp director. We pulled over and loaded T into the middle of Liz's canoe, settling her into a nest of blankets. Despite the summer heat, T was wearing a stocking cap and was wrapped in a metallic heat blanket.

Liz was incensed that the director had forced T back on the river. "She should go home, or at least back to camp."

I had a more compliant philosophy; I was just bummed there would be no more splash fights. I was starting to miss those arguments over the raisins in the granola bar.

We paddled our swaddled patient safely back to camp without further incident. To this day, Liz swears it was the hardest summer of her life.

I have many memories, stories, and friends from Camp Sunrise, as both camper and counselor. The camp helped develop me into an adult and challenged me physically, since it wasn't a camp for the disabled. I had to adapt to keep up with the kids and the counselors; there were no special rules for me. The wilderness and the river offered the perfect setting for me to find my footing.

My only regret is that Chopsaw never found Samson's glass eye in the river.

EVERGREEN

My mom drove me to college, like she had with all my siblings. I was heading to Evergreen State College in Olympia, Washington, the only school I applied for. I learned about it from my brother Greg, who had seen a Phish concert on their campus. While tripping on mushrooms, he came to the divine understanding that this was the ideal school for me.

At registration, I checked in and got my keys. I was in A Dorm, on the only drug-and alcohol-free floor. When I opened the door to my room, every flat surface was covered with empty beer cans.

My mother followed me in, saying with a sigh, "So much for drug and alcohol free."

We cleared cans and fast-food trash off my bed, started unpacking, and in stumbled a tall Japanese kid, wearing black and white plaid plastic pants, his face as red as his mohawk. He looked at me, at my mother, then reached down and picked up a warm beer from the floor and held it out to me. "Beer for you!" He bowed slightly.

I took it.

I walked my mother back to our van and gave her a big hug goodbye.

"One or two beers is okay," she said, seeing that this was already a lost cause. She later told me that she stayed and watched me amble back toward the dorm, and I never once looked back. I had come a long way from that kid at the bus stop who wanted his mom nearby, to being the kid who just wanted to get back upstairs to finish his warm beer.

The curriculum at Evergreen was as unique as the people who went there. The students could create their own courses, and there were no requirements. My brother was right. It couldn't have been more perfect for me. For example, in a traditional college, I would have had to take math courses like I had struggled with to graduate high school, but here I could pursue my interest in writing and theater. Every parent's dream.

At the end of the quarter, in lieu of grades, students filled out a comprehensive evaluation form on their own performance, the professor, and the course itself. To an outside observer, it seemed like an environment where you couldn't lose, but it was harder than you'd think. It took me days to fill these things out. I'd sit around scrutinizing what I had and had not done. I found it was easier to bullshit myself than the professor. If you didn't improve, if you didn't complete the class at a higher level than where you came in, you would get a bad evaluation from the professor. It's hard to reflect on your own growth, but these evaluations made you dig deep about what you'd actually learned, as opposed to a letter grade that doesn't reflect your unique strengths.

The class that made me fall in love with writing was called *A Sense of Place* with Bill Ransom, a published author and all-around badass. He walked on the balls of his feet like he was ready to punch someone at any moment. He confided in me that in his youth he enjoyed fighting and would let his opponents hit him two times before he would strike back. I felt like the rapport between Bill and me was more like two friends than professor and student.

Bill had a teaching style where you didn't realize you were learning. He presented material in an entertaining way, much like stand-up comedy and unlike the monotone drivel most professors spew. I took as many classes with him as he would allow.

One late autumn afternoon, I was in a creative writing seminar with Bill and thirty classmates. "I'm giving you twenty minutes to write a one-page fictional story," Bill said to the class. I didn't have a Mrs. Daniels to write for me; my scribe in college was a fellow student a few years older than me. I called her Hellcat. She had pitch-black hair to match her sense of humor. We were instant friends.

We gave Bill a nod and went into the hallway so we wouldn't disrupt the other students. We snickered as we encouraged each other in creating a horrible story about a dog catcher who would catch the dogs and fuck them in the truck with chocolate sauce as lubrication—even though we knew chocolate was bad for dogs. We were about three disturbing paragraphs in when a student poked her head out and said we were reconvening.

We took our seats on the opposite side of the circle from Bill. "Now we are going to go around the room and read our stories aloud," he said.

Hellcat's eyes popped out of her head as we both went ghostly pale and looked at each other with a weak chuckle. I tried to swallow the invisible object that was blocking my throat. Hellcat slid the notebook in front of me, implying that I was to read it. The student to Bill's left started reading his tame story. I slid the notebook back to Hellcat and pleaded with a whisper, "You read it. I can't read."

She slid it back to me and through clenched teeth whispered, "It's your story, so you better learn how, quick."

"Okay, great story. Let's hear the next one," Bill said as the ticking time bomb got closer.

I shoved the notebook back to Hellcat and hissed, "Write

something else, now!" Our turn was only four short stories away, and we were already on Bill's radar with our game of hot potato. It was clear that none of the other students had gone in an insane direction like we had.

"I like where you were going with that. Let's hear the next one," Bill said. *Tick. Tick. Tick.*

At this point, the palms of my hands were sweating, and I looked wildly around the room for an escape route. I knew if I left to go to the bathroom, Hellcat would never forgive me. The notebook sat in front of me during the next couple of stories, and I desperately read over our disaster again and again, hoping the contents had magically changed. The time bomb was ticking.

Our turn came.

"I'm curious to see what you two have come up with," Bill said with an encouraging grin.

At palsy speed, I shoved the notebook back in front of Hellcat. Like a goalie, she deflected it, bending it in half. I took the opportunity to take charge. "I have a disclaimer before she reads this story."

Hellcat's eyes fell on me with fury.

"First of all, we didn't know we were going to have to read these out loud. Secondly, some listeners may find this story to be offensively disgusting. And it is. Sorry."

Hellcat took a deep breath and flattened out the pages. "He was a man from Dayton, Ohio. Dog catching was his profession, but he did it in a very unique way…"

And then the windows of the classroom began to rattle. We all looked around, hunting for the culprit we thought was tapping on the windows. The shaking got more violent. Through the big windows I could see the giant lodgepole pines starting to roll and sway in unison, like seaweed underwater.

Someone yelled, "Earthquaaake!"

Ceiling panels started to shake loose, and everyone in the class scrambled to get under their table. Everyone but Bill. As panels fell down and dust went up, Bill calmly sat there with his hands folded on his desk. The magnitude intensified. I was on hands and knees under the table, face to face with Hellcat, and I could hear the *WOOSH* of the pine trees as the waves increased. Students screamed.

Hellcat looked me in the eye with what could have been her last words: "I'm never writing with you again."

To this day, I've thought the Earth itself couldn't handle our story and decided an earthquake would be safer.

I didn't date in high school, except for that week-long fling with the stage director. If you're differently abled in high school, most kids are not confident enough in themselves to tackle that stigma and take a chance. I had no reason to imagine that college would be any better. But I also didn't know that in college, different is unique. Different is cool, especially at Evergreen. But there was still some angst in store for me before I really began to appreciate the things that made me different.

I fell for a woman almost ten years older than me who lived down the hall. We called her Montana, after where she was from. We fooled around for a few weeks, and I thought things were moving toward a relationship when she abruptly moved to the next guy. She didn't have to move far, since the new guy happened to be my new best friend, Hal. I was heartbroken. I didn't handle it well, going so far as to chase Hal with my Senegalese machete.

One Thursday evening in November, I was pouting in my room, lying in bed in the dark. It was way too early for a college student to be in bed. There was a rapid knock at my door and before I could tell them to fuck off, the two people I was trying to avoid burst in with an explosion of harsh light.

Montana said, "We need your help with Crazy Jim!"

"You need to hold him down," Hal added.

Crazy Jim lived on the floor below us. He was in his late twenties and a chess master. He had long hair, a wild, unkempt beard, and a glazed, faraway look, like he was perpetually tripping on acid. He spoke with a cosmic cadence: odd pauses. And words…trickling out…two or three…at a time.

I worried Crazy Jim must have finally snapped. I jumped up, pulled on my fleece pants, and followed them out of my cavern of self-pity.

Hal and Montana led me to our repulsive community kitchen, where I found Jim pacing. I had been psyching myself up to tackle him, but he seemed his normal eccentric self. He didn't have a butcher knife to anyone's throat, and he wasn't spurting blood.

I looked around for an explanation and locked eyes with Montana. My little '90s heart broke all over again when I realized she was wearing a black, shoulder-length wig like Uma Thurman in *Pulp Fiction*.

"Jim needs us for a favor," she said.

Jim cut in, "I have chosen…you to help me…with this. The strong men…must forcibly…hold me down…while…this beautiful woman rids me…of my facial hair." He was chillingly serious. Only Crazy Jim could make a beard trim terrifying.

Montana nervously adjusted her wig.

As Jim laid down the guidelines, more people stumbled into

the kitchen, many of them drunk. An eager audience. Jim elaborated, "I haven't shaved...for seven years. I made...a pact with myself never...to do it again. This is the only way...it can happen."

A lump formed in my stomach.

"I want all...the hair that is taken...from my face...to be gathered up and...saved. No one is allowed...to steal any."

"Who would steal someone else's facial hair?" I whispered to Hal.

"You have...half an hour to prepare," Jim told us. "I'm going to shower...and ready my body...for the ritual...Find some restraints...to tie me down with."

He left the kitchen and headed to his room on the eighth floor.

"What kind of bullshit did you guys get me into?" I asked.

"I'm going to go get my bike lock," Montana replied.

Hal and I prepared the ceremonial throne. One of the spectators offered up a roll of duct tape, and we fastened a chair to the ninth floor balcony rail, with my heart racing and my hands shaking more than usual. Word spread through the dorm, and the crowd grew. Montana returned with the cable lock and rubbed Hal's back to let him know she was there. Watching the two of them flirt while they worked made my teeth audibly grind. They didn't seem to notice, or if they did, they didn't care.

"Um, Hal," I said.

They both looked up.

"Do you think he'll fight back?"

"Are you asking if you should get your machete?" Hal asked, and together with Montana immediately answered, "No!"

Someone came up from the eighth floor with clippers, shaving cream, and a straight-edge razor. "Jim sent these up for you to familiarize yourselves with."

The door to the stairwell banged open, and Jim walked out onto the balcony, dripping wet, wearing nothing but purple tighty-whities and red and green warpaint. He was followed by an entourage of drunk women from the eighth floor. The crowd went silent. Jim walked to the chair and sat down. He looked around. Then, with his right hand, he pulled the elastic waistband of his underwear away from his body and fished around with his left hand. "I need someone…to go down and get…the rope…from my room."

Happy for any chance to get away, I said, "I'll go," and bolted for the door.

"You'll need…my keys," he said, pulling them out from his Jockeys.

I looked at Montana. "Maybe you should go."

She gave me a very clear the-fuck-I-am look.

I held my breath and grabbed the warm keys. At least they weren't wet.

Hal began taping Jim's arm to the railing.

Jim hissed after me, "Don't let…anyone in my room."

"No worries, Jim," I said over my shoulder. "No worries."

I ran down the stairs and when I got to his room, I picked through his keys, forced to touch each one until I found the one that opened the door. Inside, I found a plastic bag filled with leather straps and fifty feet of coiled rope. As I was leaving, three drunk students stumbled in and plopped themselves down on the floor.

Back upstairs, Jim sat with his arms out to either side, crucifix-style, and taped securely to the railing. "Did anyone try…to get in my room?" he asked.

"No," I lied. "What do you want me to do with your keys?"

He nodded toward his crotch. "I want them...back...where you found them."

I didn't know Jim that well and didn't plan on knowing him for much longer. "Would it be okay if I just put them between your legs?" I said, tossing them more than a little unkindly onto his nuts without waiting for a reply. He winced and tested the strength of the tape job. Luckily, it held.

Kneeling in front of Jim, Hal and Montana tentatively taped his bare, hairy legs to the chair. Crazy Jim had zero reservations about his bare skin being duct-taped, really living up to his nickname.

"I will be fighting back now," Jim said with startling clarity. He gave a mighty heave, and both legs broke free. I bent down to grab one of them, and he kicked me square in the chest. I fell back on my ass into the midst of the awestruck crowd. I decided to up my dedication to this project and grabbed the rope. One of the spectators stepped forward and caught the other of Jim's pale, flailing legs, and they held it down. I had experience with ropes from Camp Sunrise and put it to the test, trussing up Jim's ankles tightly, like a natural calf-roper.

Jim was snorting and spitting, whipping his greasy, wet ponytail like a scorpion's tail. Another man was trying to control his writhing torso, as the warpaint smeared on his clothes. Jim groaned as I pulled the rope tight and tied the other end to the railing. In a gentler tone, he asked me, "Could we...loosen the rope...a little bit?"

"Not right now," I said, rubbing my chest. "Maybe after you cool down."

We checked all our knots and restraints and finished off by wrapping Montana's bicycle lock around his chest and locking it behind the chair. I sidebarred with Hal as we dodged the whipping ponytail, and we decided to each put an arm under one of Jim's armpits, through the bars of the railing behind him, and then grasp each other's wrist. This would leave us with a free arm for any shenanigans Jim had coming.

Jim's head was still rocking around. I grabbed his slippery ponytail with my free hand and yanked back as hard as I could.

"We're in place," Hal told Montana.

We had our backs to Montana and the crowd. She stepped forward, the clippers buzzing. Jim started to shake like he was possessed, and I kept expecting his head to spin around. The blaze of lunacy in his eyes was matched by Montana's terror.

The tiny motor in the clippers labored as Montana mowed through the gnarled tangles of Jim's beard. Suddenly, there was a fire crackling close to my ear and the smell of burning hair. A lighter was pulled away as a fire grew on Jim's face. His friend Brian had come forward out of the crowd and now stood back, BIC in hand. Montana pummeled at the flames with her free hand, but as soon as it was out, Brian was back with his lighter, igniting it once again.

"Stop!" Montana shrieked.

This had escalated to a new flammable level, and I was starting to worry campus police might soon be on the scene.

"Let it burn," Jim growled. Of course he had set up this insane backup plan.

"Put that shit out!" I shouted at Brian. "You're gonna catch *my* hair on fire!"

Montana smacked out the fire.

The crowd started chanting, "Je-sus-Jim! Je-sus-Jim!"

I felt nauseous. I wasn't sure if it was the smell of charred hair, the chanting, or Jim snorting and spitting flecks of foam like a racehorse with rabies. *Am I in a cult?*

The clippers stopped, but the chanting didn't.

"That's as close as I can get with these," said Montana, as she traded the clippers to the crowd for a razor and shaving cream. Jim's face was now blotchy and reddened from the fire and smacking.

I looked at Hal, and we reminded each other to breathe. Jim stopped struggling and asked us if we could loosen our hold on his shoulders.

"Are you gonna be a good boy?" I replied. The tone of his growl let me know he was, so I eased up my grip a little.

Montana was ready for the finale: the close shave. She spread a thick layer of shaving cream on Jim's face with surprising gentleness, then brought the razor up. She had been scared through the entire ordeal, but now it was clear she had never shaved anyone, let alone a werewolf.

"Stay still," Hal said to Jim. "Or she's gonna cut you."

"He's right," Montana added.

Jim said, "It would be very…beneficial to this project…if I didn't end up with…any permanent scars."

The chanting grew hushed as Montana took her first swipe.

"Hold the razor down," a backseat shaver yelled from the crowd, "not up."

"He's right," Hal said.

Montana proceeded to shave Jim without so much as a nick. Hal and I relaxed our hold. The prophecy had been fulfilled. Montana stepped away, and someone dumped a bucket of cold water over Jim's head. His warpaint streaked down his chest toward his keys, turning his tighty-whities tie-dyed.

Hal and I stepped back next to Montana to admire our work, a soaking warrior taped to a cold, metal crucifix. "Good job," I told Montana.

"Yeah," she said. "He looks handsome without a beard."

I turned to the crowd. "What would you guys think if we left Jim here for a while?"

They cheered.

"That was not part of the arrangement," Jim snarled, glaring up at us.

We untied his legs first. Suddenly, he tried with all his might to break the tape from his arms, like a much smaller King Kong. The tape held but reignited the furnace of rage in his eyes. I never saw so many drunk people scatter all at once. I was halfway to the door myself before I steeled myself and went back to join Hal. It was time to free the beast.

I cut Jim's arms free with a knife, then we ripped the tape off, taking patches of hair with it. Jim stood up and rubbed his wrists. He grabbed his keys and put them back where he thought they belonged. Someone handed him a dustpan and a broom. He mushed his wet hair into a pile and shoved it into a Ziploc. "Is this all of it?" he asked with grave intensity.

I picked some of his singed hair out of my own goatee and handed it to him. "This should be all of it."

Jim shook hands and thanked us, as if we had just completed some extremely normal transaction. He invited us down to his place for celebratory drinks, then turned and walked away, leaving me with the girl who had dumped me for my best friend, and a paint-streaked chair still taped to the railing.

I started doing stand-up my junior year. You don't become a comedian the moment you start doing stand-up, but my journey started here. I had always been a joker at heart and inflicted my humor on friends and family members, but this was my first foray in front of a willing audience. There was an open-mic night in the housing community center on campus every Tuesday; I had been going there to watch slam poetry, singers and songwriters since my freshman year. Nobody was doing stand-up.

I hesitated to tell my friends that I thought I could be funny up there and, after three weeks of chickening out, I jumped off the ledge. I told the guy in charge to put my name on the list and warned him that he was probably going to have to physically force me onstage.

I had ten minutes to perform. If you're not familiar with open-mic comedy, ten minutes is an eternity for a virgin comedian. I had already been on campus for two years, so most everyone was familiar with the way I moved, which helped disguise my nervous jitters. I clumsily wrestled the mic from the stand, then dragged a bulky wooden chair over and promptly sat down, thereby breaking the first rule of stand-up comedy: standing up. I don't even think I mentioned palsy in my set, which is something I quickly learned to always do: I have to address the crippled elephant in the room to make the audience feel comfortable. For my first comedy set, I told stories about my experiences as Chopsaw, the camp counselor, and life in Africa. People listened and laughed when they were supposed to, and when I got that first laugh, a huge amount of pressure lifted. *This isn't a huge mistake.* At the end of my set, I felt confident enough to tell the audience that I'd be back the next week. When I came offstage, I was buzzing with a newfound energy.

I spent that week thinking about what I would talk about onstage in my next performance, while spreading the word to anyone who would listen that I was now a stand-up comedian. That first show there were twenty people in the audience. The next week there were fifty, and most of them left after my set. It seemed they were there to see this oddity.

I did the open mic four weeks in a row to steadily growing audiences, and on the fourth go-round, I ate shit like a plow horse. For me, bombing feels like my soul is being sucked out of my anus with a plunger. The audience wasn't laughing, and my cadence and connection with them were gone. Perhaps they saw me as I truly was: a young comic getting ahead of himself, thinking he was hotshot right out of the gates. *How dare you waste our time with this charade? You think this is entertaining?* Looking back today, after experiencing a genuine bomb, I realize that show was more of a bump in the road. Regardless, the show was awful. I moped around for days. I didn't understand it at the time, but that's how it's supposed to go—you're supposed to eat a little shit every now and again to remind you not to eat shit at all.

One day, while still moping around on campus, wondering if it was too late to become an accountant, an older student inquired why I was not my usual cheerful self.

"I bombed trying to do stand-up."

He gasped. "Wow, I did stand-up for many years! That's a cutthroat business."

"It is?"

"Oh yeah," he replied. "There's nothing harder to do than to stand alone and be funny on command in front of strangers. You have to make your personal experiences relatable to them so they can laugh. And bombing is just part of it."

Hearing this excited me and inspired me to get back onstage. I had already experienced some success. I had seen growth in the size of my audience week after week; now I just had to find stronger ways to connect with them.

In my senior year, I changed my academic focus from writing to theater. Plugging away at the open mic had shown me a whole new medium for my creativity, and it was one for which I didn't need a Hellcat or Mrs. Daniels. All of my comedy was flowing directly out of my mind; I didn't write anything down, and I still don't.

Students came to theater from all angles. There were stage managers, actors, playwrights, and then kids like me, trying to figure something out so we didn't have to get a day job.

In my class called The Empty Stage, we performed Georg Büchner's play *Danton's Death*, in which I was cast in such memorable roles as Citizen 4 and Prisoner 2. The week after the final performance, back in class, the professor told us with a laugh that his wife enjoyed the play, particularly the young man who was so talented as to play such a convincing paraplegic. He looked pointedly at me as the class laughed. Not only did this hurt my feelings, it was a brutal eye-opener. People weren't seeing me act as Prisoner 2, they were only seeing palsy boy Blue.

One of our assignments had us choose between writing and directing a play, or to act in another student's production. I came up with the idea to do stand-up with actors. As I got into certain bits, the actors would come onstage, and I would step away from the mic and become part of the scene. When each sketch ended, I stepped back up to the mic to do more stand-up. We practiced maybe four times. I told the actors I had no idea what bits I would be doing between the planned sketches and to just listen for their cue.

The performance went surprisingly well, considering the lack of preparation. The feedback I took from the professor was, "You directed your cast very well. The thing you need to work on is yourself. You can move around all you want when you're doing the set-up, but when it comes to the punchline, you need to plant yourself and say it like you mean it."

Since then, I've become more aware of my own body language and placement onstage.

After The Empty Stage finished, I had one semester of school left before my release into the wild. For my final credits, I decided to study motivational speaking and stand-up comedy. This idea was put into my head by an Evergreen staff member named Linda Pickering, a no-nonsense woman who had endured my sarcastic sense of humor for the past four years. She ran the campus's Access Services office, which provided alternative study options to students with physical and mental disabilities.

As much as I've always enjoyed creative writing, the actual physical side of it is a struggle. My eyes have a hard time focusing on the letters on the screen, and my fingers rarely hit the right keys. Between my horrible spelling and my scattershot typing, spellcheck can't find the correct, or any English word, to suggest.

Every semester I'd choose a student to assist me, and Linda noticed a pattern where I'd pick the cutest girls as notetakers and would often hook up with them. Linda said, "Josh, you realize that this is not a personal dating service?"

"Well, I just have a gift, Linda. What can I do?"

She once told me there were eight people attending Evergreen who had multiple personalities. My response was, "I think I dated at least twelve of them."

Linda had a treasure trove of performances on VHS, featuring different flavors of disabilities being displayed in beautiful ways. From ballet dancers in wheelchairs to blind poets and authors, I was amazed to see so many people not just overcoming, but also thriving in the bodies they were given. Through this, I also realized being disabled is the largest minority group in the world. It's also the only minority group you can join at any time.

One of the tapes in Linda's hodgepodge library featured professional comedians with disabilities. Growing up, the comics who impressed me most were the ones who broke down barriers; Richard Pryor did it with race, Ellen DeGeneres did it with homosexuality. I was amazed to discover there were comedians out there doing the same thing with disabilities. I wasn't blazing a trail; I was ambling down this path that others had already hacked their way through, or more accurately, painstakingly pushed their wheelchairs through. It was reassuring to know I wasn't the only one on that trail.

Those tapes introduced me to Kathy Buckley, Brett Leake, and Chris Fonseca. Kathy Buckley is deaf and was run over by a Jeep. She hurdled both of those challenges to become a hilarious comic and motivational speaker. Brett Leake has multiple sclerosis, and seeing him perform on *The Tonight Show* was the first time I had ever seen someone with a disability on late night TV. The comic who really hit home for me was Chris Fonseca.

Chris has severe cerebral palsy and performs from a wheelchair. His speech is slow and labored, and his audience hangs on every word, because he's a master of his craft; he's unafraid to be himself, to create his own style of impeccable timing. More than that, he talks about his real life and his disability. I realized I could do that, too. He's been tremendously successful, with appearances on *The Late Show* with David Letterman and *Baywatch*. He made me realize, for the first time, that a career in stand-up comedy could actually be an option for me.

BACK TO AFRICA

In my junior year of college, I returned to Senegal by myself. It was my first solo international flight. A tall man with a limp and a cane picked me up at the Dakar airport. In the car, he smiled a lot and tested my rusty Wolof. I was here to intern at the Hann Forest and Zoological Park, or as the locals called it, the Parc de Hann zoo. Eager to learn as much as possible, I asked him what I might expect from the job.

"Hey, I'm just the driver, man."

The sun beat on the sandy blacktop as the car shook, rattled, and vibrated, swerving around herds of goats and peanut vendors. The thick smell of the ocean saturated everything. Everyone's clothing was a collection of vibrant patterns that would make a parrot swoon. I greedily absorbed as much as I could. It had been two years since I had last been here; it felt right to be back in my second home.

At the gates of the Parc de Hann zoo, guards with rifles saluted us as we rolled in, then looked again to take in the toubab with disheveled long blonde hair in the back seat. I stared back, wondering if these serious guns were to protect the people from the animals or vice versa. Part of me was hoping it was a Jurassic Park situation. The car followed the beaten ruts to the sandy yard where the Ndiayes lived, my host family for the next three months. I struggled out of the car and stretched my well-traveled, crooked body as the chauffeur leaned on the horn. The faces of three eager young boys popped up from behind the fence of bougainvillea. From their raised eyebrows and whispers, I could tell I was not what they were expecting.

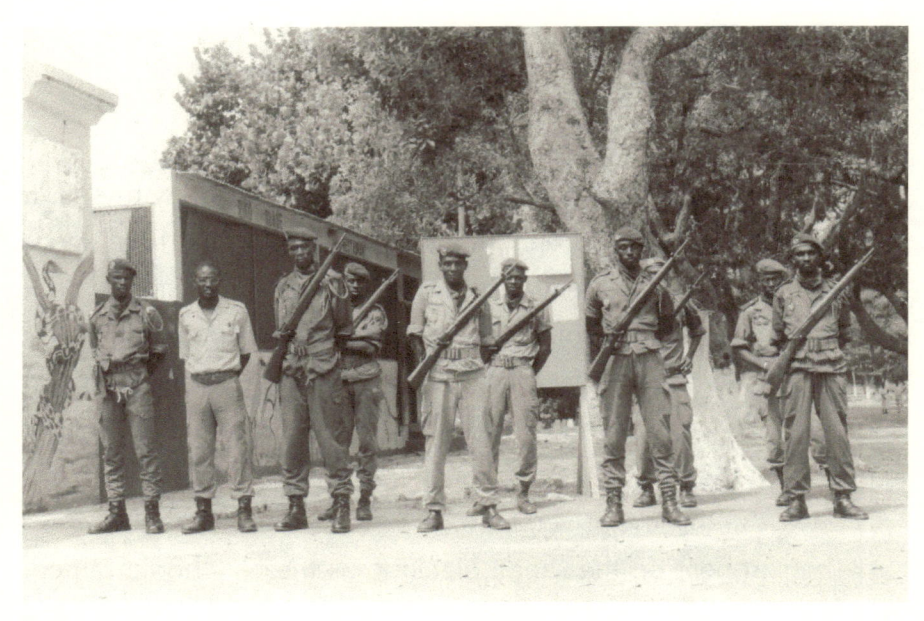

The no-nonsense guards of Parc de Haan zoo.

A thick-framed man stepped out, dressed in what appeared to be a general's uniform complete with medals and accented with a glinting revolver in a leather holster on his belt. He had a long face with a graying mustache and close-cut hair. His shiny black shoes sunk into the sand. He said something in Wolof to the boys in the yard, and they followed close on his heels. *Is this a military zoo? What have I gotten myself into?*

"I am Abu Ndiaye," the decorated man said in French, extending his hand.

"My name is Bamba Djot," I said in Wolof.

"Djot is a bad last name," he said with a smile.

"Ndiaye eat rice until they die," I replied in Wolof with a bigger smile. There are relatively few last names in Wolof, and many of them have playful rivalries. The Djots and the Ndiayes had a playful animosity toward one another, and my knowledge of this rivalry put the family at ease.

Mr. Ndiaye introduced the three boys: the oldest Papis, the next Sheikh, and then Malik. I didn't remember their names till much later, but they all shyly shook my tangled right hand. I soon discovered Mr. Ndiaye was the head of security for the zoo, which explained his extreme dress code.

"I can't have a Djot stay at my house. You are now officially a Ndiaye."

I accepted the honor and followed the chauffeur back to the trunk to grab my bags.

Mr. Ndiaye insisted the boys take them for me. "Is your leg sick?" he asked.

"No, it's just like that."

It was never mentioned again.

The tall chauffeur shook my hand and bid me good day. I thanked him and followed the Ndiayes through the wooden door into my new home. The concrete floor was cool. My little brothers struggled under the weight of my bags, which were mostly filled with gifts from the States for the family. There were Minnesota sweets and clothing, and the cherry on top: a pristine soccer ball.

They brought me into a large room with high ceilings. The walls were smooth for the most part and painted a dirty blue. There was a queen-size bed with mosquito netting hung above it, which reminded me to take a malaria pill. I tried chatting with the boys in French but soon realized that my high school French was better than their elementary school French, so we were going to have to rely on Wolof, hand gestures, and grunting—the true universal language.

I opened the wooden shutters in my room to let more of Africa in. Women's voices carried with the wind. I saw them come around the corner into the yard: two tall, skinny girls, and one shorter, stout girl, all looking about the age of 20. I had trouble guessing Senegalese women's ages; the 12-year-olds looked like they were 20, and the 45-year-olds also looked like they were 20.

"*Ana toubab bi?*" one of the women asked Sheikh. *Where is the White man?*

It was nice being back in Senegal, where being White meant you were the odd man out. And being White and disabled meant I was the oddest man out.

Over dinner of rice and fish, I met the rest of the family. We sat on the floor and ate with our hands from one big platter. I called Mrs. Ndiaye *Yahy*, which conveniently enough means mother in Wolof. She was very welcoming and kind to her new, strange son. Yahy spent her days as a high school geography teacher. The young women—who I had eavesdropped on talking to the boys—were their sister, a cousin, and the shorter, stout one was their maid. They peppered me with questions about my life, especially my cerebral palsy. In Senegal, as with many Islamic countries, you eat with your right hand, and your left is saved for bathroom business. My left has both jobs, so the family offered me a spoon.

I went to bed early, jet lag and all. Tired as I was, I swear I had a smile on my face. Tucked in my mosquito net fortress, I slept heavily into the middle of the night when I was pulled awake by the cliché pounding of rain on a tin roof. I know everyone talks about it on their travels to the third world, but there is something to it. I'd never been in a real African rainstorm, at least not to my memory. The pounding sounded like someone shaking a bag of seashells. All the rain gave me the sudden cruel realization that I had no idea where the bathroom was. In all my excitement, I hadn't peed since I'd gotten off the plane.

I wasn't about to go stumbling around in the dark house; the image of Mr. Ndiaye's handgun came to mind. What if he thought I was a burglar? Could I climb up and pee out the high window? And if Mr. Ndiaye caught me doing that, would he shoot me anyway? *Don't shoot, this is how we do it in America, promise!*

There was no door to my room, only a thin, red piece of African cloth. A light came on, and I saw Mr. Ndiaye wearing no shirt, just black Adidas workout pants and flip-flops, bustling about, putting down pots and pans to catch the renegade raindrops. I was relieved to see there was no gun on his hip. I got up, but I couldn't remember how to say pee in Wolof, so I did the universal pee pee dance. He was a little surprised to see me up, and I noticed the rest of the family was now awake and battening down the hatches.

"Bamba, *bëgëna saw?*" he asked.

Saw, saw, that's it. I nodded yes.

He pointed to the door, where I could hear the rain pounding against it. "Just stand in the doorway and pee out on the front steps."

"Okay."

"Lock the door when you're done and turn off the lights."

All the pots and pans were in place, and each made a different plinking sound, like a tiny reggae band playing their steel drums. The family said goodnight again. While I was relieving myself, I heard the boys giggling behind me. Guess I could have gone out the window after all.

After locking the door and turning out the lights, I lay in my bed wide-awake for hours, consumed by jet lag. When the morning finally came, I found out there wasn't any bathroom in the house. You had to go next door to use a hole in the ground or to take a shower. When you went to the bathroom, not only did your family know, but the neighbors did as well.

A week passed as I adjusted to my new family and the scary hole next door. Late one night, I was sweating peacefully in bed when I awoke to a dark figure untucking the mosquito net. The tall, skinny man sat on the edge of the bed and slapped the sand off the bottoms of his feet before crawling in next to me, lying down, and immediately going to sleep. I laid awake into the night, wondering who my new bedmate was. The bed was just big enough so we could each have our own, narrow side.

In the morning, over fresh baguette and sugary coffee water, I asked, "Who is that?" gesturing through the red curtain of my doorway, toward the slumbering body in what I thought was *my* bed.

"That's Sheikh Omar, your uncle," said Mr. Ndiaye.

It turned out that room was his, and it was probably weirder for him to encounter me—a contorted White guy, snoring in *his* bed. Later in the afternoon, after I got home from working at the zoo, I shook hands with my new uncle. He had a serious face and well-kept fingernails, and only dressed in army fatigues. He was a night watchman at the zoo and worked strange hours. He always got home in the middle of the night and dutifully climbed over me into bed like we were an old married couple.

From then on, the nights were long; the body heat multiplied by two, but the hornbills and fire finches chirped me awake every sunrise regardless of how little sleep I got. I always woke up dehydrated from sweating gallons every night, the muggy heat and sticky skin clinging to our sheet. I had finally acclimated to sleeping next to grown-ass Uncle Omar when I woke to discover I had become an Oreo. Sheikh Omar was to my left, and a new mystery man was to my right. He was shorter than Omar but had a thicker frame. Suddenly, I was conscious of space, color, and gender. Back in the States, the idea of sharing a bed with two uncles is unheard of, and in fact rather frowned upon. But in Africa, if you have even a sliver of real estate in your bed, the more the merrier.

This new Uncle Jaga was studying English at the university. He was much friendlier than Sheikh Omar; we talked in Wolof, French, and English. "What time is it?" was his best English phrase. "It's time for you to get a watch," was my favorite reply. After some explaining, he thought this was rather funny.

If only he could see how far my comedy has come since then.

Late one night, one of my bed uncles let in a cockroach to share our warmth. It crawled through the thicket of my chest hair, pausing on my sternum to check its map. My groggy calculations told me that a cockroach plus a closed mosquito net equaled a long night of scurrying back and forth over us. I thought back to my old, trusted friend the roach-wrecking billy club and wished I had it now. I could feel each of the six legs, like toothpicks, dancing on my skin. My left hand snapped up like a praying mantis and grabbed the roach between my thumb and index finger, crushing it. I threw it in Sheikh Omar's direction and drifted back to sleep. My uncles were gone before I woke up, but the roach was there, on its back, two legs still twitching.

The roaches were the least of my bug problems. At night the walls were blanketed with mosquitoes, and despite the netting, I got bit and contracted malaria. I was as sick as I had ever been.

My entire body was so sore, it felt like I had fallen from a four-story building and then been promptly hit by a Mack truck. Every joint was in unimaginable pain, and I had a boiling fever to top it off. My uncles slept elsewhere those nights, perhaps worried they'd wake up next to my crippled corpse. My adopted family was clearly concerned for me, but they didn't have the bedside manner I missed from my mother.

After four days of delirium and a 106-degree fever, my host family handed me off to a friend of my father's, who took me by cab to see a doctor who practiced western medicine. He gave me a series of shots in my butt and pills for the pain. Within two days, I was back on my feet.

Shortly after that, I was moved into the boys' room. I had my own bed but no mosquito net because I had already had malaria. My three younger brothers shared a pad on the floor. I felt like a camp counselor all over again.

Malik had a problem with wetting the bed. On a nightly basis, out of self-preservation, his older brothers would slap him awake, "Get up and go!" Seeing as there was no toilet in the house, the boys peed in a purple bucket in our room several times during the course of a night. Little Malik had trouble hitting his target, and the sound of urine sporadically falling in a bucket was quite a way to wake up.

And then *I* would have to pee. There's something about a young White man in the middle of an African night trying to tinkle quietly into a bucket. I think my aim was even worse than Malik's.

I stayed in that room the remainder of my being a Ndiaye. The strong smell of piss in a bucket from four people was my regular wake-up call. I had no problem jumping up and getting ready for work, trading the stench of that bucket for the stink of the zoo.

◯◯◯

Parc de Hann zoo was small by American standards, and well-worn. All the cages' bars were painted turquoise, faded and chipped away by wear and tear from the animals. There were seven zookeepers, and although I was assigned an internship with Pop, I spent an equal amount of time with Usman, who was friendly and playful, with a constant smile on his bald, round head. He would seek me out whenever I was working to joke around. Like at my host home, Wolof and French were the only languages spoken.

In my three months at Parc de Hann, I became quite knowledgeable about the animals I was interested in. I can't tell you shit about a fish eagle, but I can tell you that a female hyena has a mock penis. My duties at the zoo were many: hosing the cages, feeding the animals, weeding, sweeping sidewalks, and general monkey boy for the real zookeeper. I would also take it upon myself to give tours to the occasional English speakers that came through.

I shadowed Usman every day, even though he wasn't technically the zookeeper I was assigned to. Built like a cinder block, his arms were bigger in diameter than the zoo's twelve-foot python. He knew every animal in the zoo, and what it was thinking. I looked up to him. He was one of the only zookeepers who truly respected the animals. He had two terrifying scars on his wrist. After a month, I got the courage to ask him what happened.

He explained that several years before, the biggest male baboon in the zoo had escaped. The other keepers always went to Usman to catch the monkeys. He got a sweet potato—which he knew was this guy's favorite—and coaxed the baboon close, grabbed it gently by its wrist, and pulled him onto his lap. Usman said everything was fine, crisis averted, until some little kids came over to check it out, and another male baboon called out a challenge. The baboon on Usman's lap freaked. It turned like lightning and sunk its two-inch fangs into Usman's wrist, slicing the major arteries and almost severing his hand. In self-defense, Usman snapped out with his other hand and crushed the baboon's throat, killing it instantly.

His boss—my host father Abu—cried as he drove Usman to the hospital. Usman missed work for three months. He teared up at the memory and confessed he still felt bad for killing the animal. I hoped that I wouldn't ever have to palsy punch a primate.

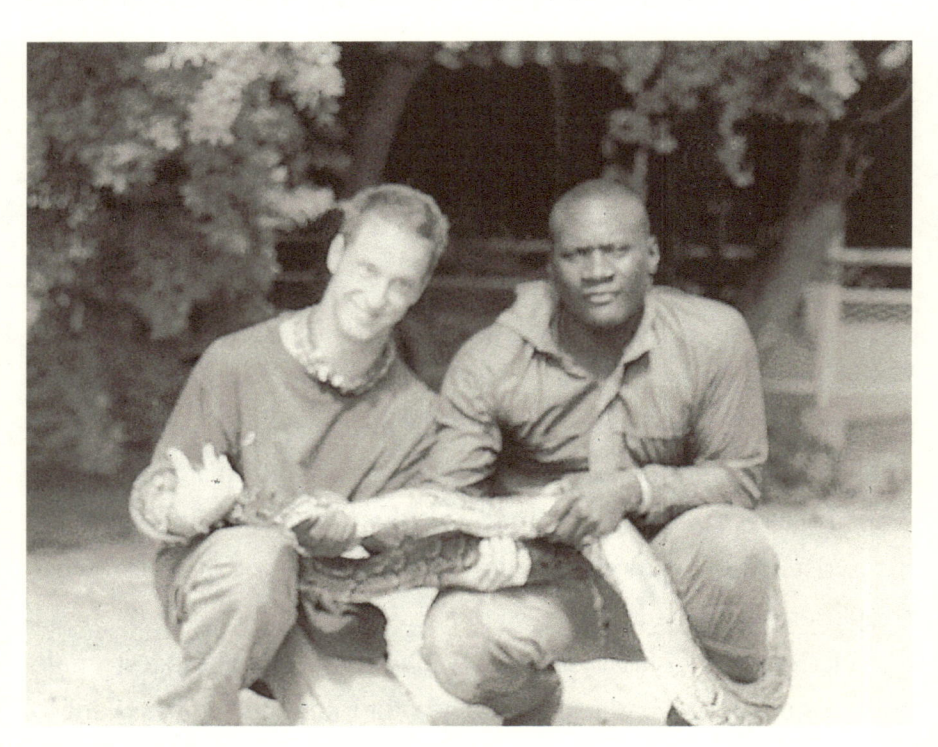

Me and Usman with a big-ass python.

Usman had an extraordinary way with all the animals. Almost every creature acted differently with him than they did with the other zookeepers. He would leap over guardrails effortlessly; he had his massive keyring memorized and the locks and keys snapped together like magnets. He would talk in low tones to whatever beast was on the other side of the bars, and each language was different and specific to that animal. There was a throaty *coo* for the big cats, and a strange *chuk chuk chuk* sound to get the ornery honey badger's attention.

I'd seen him climb fearlessly into cages with hyenas, crocodiles, and venomous snakes, but on this particular day Usman was hopping the rail to a large female lion's enclosure. He'd known this lioness for her entire life: She had been born at the zoo, and he had named her Fatou. I felt sad for her, separated from the rest of the lions, in a cage no bigger than five feet by eight feet.

"Fatou is very friendly and playful," Usman said, as he beckoned me to climb over the guardrail and approach the weathered bars.

My heart kicked up, and I pretended I wasn't terrified—I heard they can smell fear. Usman's infectious smile put me at ease. I moved my hands between the bars and patted her solid head. She was smaller than our big mountain lion, but much thicker. She purred as I scratched behind her ear and brushed away the flies that were always picking away at the animals.

When I was making my rounds the next day, I approached Fatou's cage. As she leapt from one end to the other, I could see how much power was contained in her small cell. The poor thing was so lonely. She playfully bounded up, remembering me from the day before. I clambered over the guardrail to scratch my new friend behind her ears, as I had seen Usman do. A young girl tentatively approached the rail to watch what this toubab was up to.

I came right up to the bars, and Fatou reared up on her hind legs, stretching against the bars. She was surprisingly taller than me and showing it off. I thought I caught a twinge of something, a change in her eye; something that reminded me that even though she was born in captivity, she was still the queen of the jungle. But then she dropped down on all fours and pushed the side of her face and shoulder into the bars. She rubbed along them and rumbled a deep, bass purr I could feel in my chest.

Fatou walked back and forth like this, turning herself once again into a giant house cat. I petted her once, twice, and on the third time, she snapped into the apex predator she really was. As if in slow motion, her leg came up over her head between the bars, each toe spread apart and every two-inch, yellowish claw forever ingrained in my brain. I could see every sinewy muscle tighten as her paw came down like a spiked baseball bat, hitting me on the wrist.

My lightning palsy reflexes saved my life as I sprang away from the bars. I don't remember jumping the guardrail. I looked at my wrist. No pain or blood. There was also no sign of the girl, who to this day probably tells people about the toubab who mistook a lion for a house cat.

The tension in the air was thick, and it was deathly quiet. I looked around to find every animal in the zoo staring directly into my primal soul. I realized how connected we were and that if we were in the Serengeti right now, there would be a feeding frenzy, with me as the main course. The nearby hyenas stared at me with a look that suggested, *hey come try that with us.*

Upon closer inspection, I located a small wound. One claw had hit me and taken out a perfect little triangle of meat on my inner wrist, nearly nailing an artery. Through the tiny hole, I could see down to the bone. It never bled, which was somehow more disturbing than if it had been a bloody mess. I hid it from everyone as long as I could, especially Usman. I felt like I had let him down. I was embarrassed by my stupidity to think that I could suddenly jump into his experienced boots.

But of course, word of my foolishness spread throughout the zoo. The other keepers teased me, and that wasn't the end of it. When Mrs. Ndiaye found out, she smacked me and cursed me out in only the way a mother can.

Usman roasted me the most. "Want to get into the crocodile cage next?"

"*Mayma sama jàm,*" I replied. *Give me my peace.*

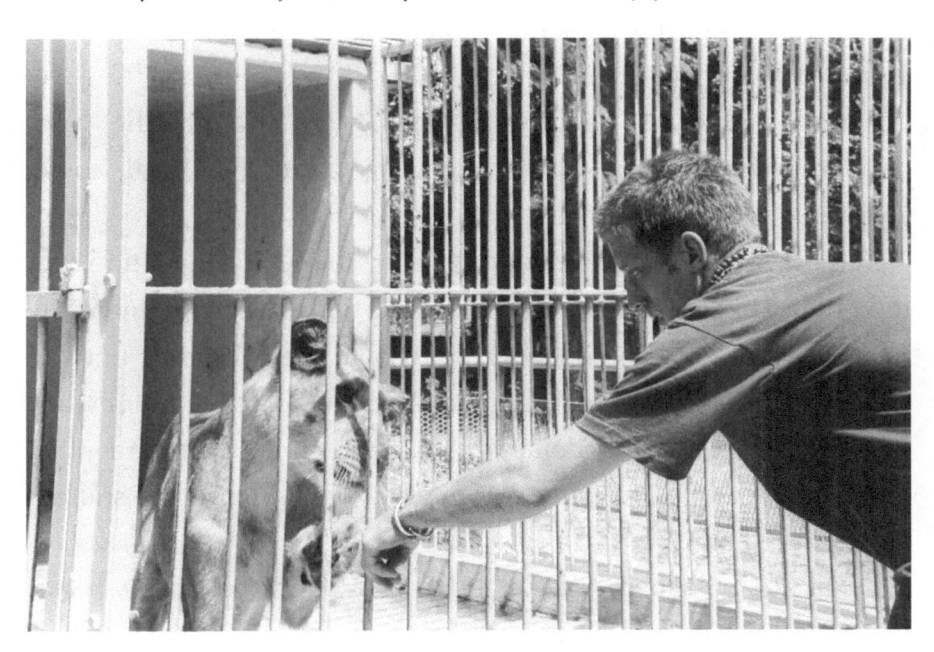

Me with Fatou, the lioness who punctured me.

I was nearing the end of my stay when I was asked to give a tour to a woman from Detroit. I was excited to speak English with another American and to show off my zoo skills. The guest was a young African-American woman visiting for the Peace Corps. She clearly did not know what to make of this wobbly, wild-haired toubab as her tour guide. It seemed she would be more comfortable if I were on the other side of the bars.

First stop, the mountain lions. I casually jumped over the guardrail and confidently approached their cage. I clicked my tongue to let them know I was here. Of all the big cats, they were the ones I spent the most time with; they really seemed like giant house cats. They bounded over to me, rubbing their heads against the bars, purring as I scratched them and licking me with their sandpaper tongues.

I looked at the visitor, expecting her to be impressed, and she was anything but. The look on her face said, *I came to Africa to get away from goofy White bullshit.*

Nonetheless, I eagerly dragged her through the zoo, peppering her with awkward questions about life back home: "Does pizza still taste good?"

The last stop on the Amazing Josh Blue Zoo Adventure was the chimpanzees. One of the chimps, a four-year-old named Tali, had been born in captivity and raised by a French family until he was two. The family quickly realized they couldn't keep him when he could reach the chandelier with a single jump. Not to mention the fact that a chimp is strong enough to handily beat the shit out of an entire family.

Tali was bilingual—French and Chimp—and knew a few tricks. He could wash his hands, jump and clap on command, and he'd give you a kiss if you asked him really nicely: *"Donne-moi un baiser."*

I jumped over the guardrail and walked up to the bars. Tali and I went through our routine, doing our tricks, building up to the grand finale of the kiss on the lips. That would surely impress my guest. "Tali," I said, "donne-moi un baiser."

Tali ignored me. Cold shoulder, in fact.

"Come on. Donne-moi un baiser."

Tali turned to me and leaned in, so I leaned in for the kiss. Like lightning, his arms shot out. I could hear the noise of coarse hair squeezing through the bars. He locked his hands behind my neck and, in the same motion, jumped up, grabbed the bars below with his feet, and pulled in as hard as he possibly could. My face slammed against the cage, and the sound was like a watermelon falling on a cold concrete floor.

Just as quickly as he had tricked me, Tali let go and retreated to the back of his cage. Lucky for me. My nose narrowly missed being broken, and he could have hammered my head into the cage fifteen times, turning my skull into mush if he wanted to. When my brain cleared, I was still holding the bars to steady myself.

I waved away the cartoon birds over my head and turned to look at the visitor to make sure she was still enjoying her zoo experience. She finally seemed entertained.

"Man! You got fucked up!"

The blood trickling down my face signaled this was the end of the tour. The woman walked off, but Usman had witnessed the entire scene. He came over and beckoned me to come back to the bars on Tali's cage. I balked; one head smash per day was enough for me. Usman, being the alpha primate, reassured me that I was safe, and I tentatively walked back over. He turned to Tali like a furious father. "Apologize! Look what you did!"

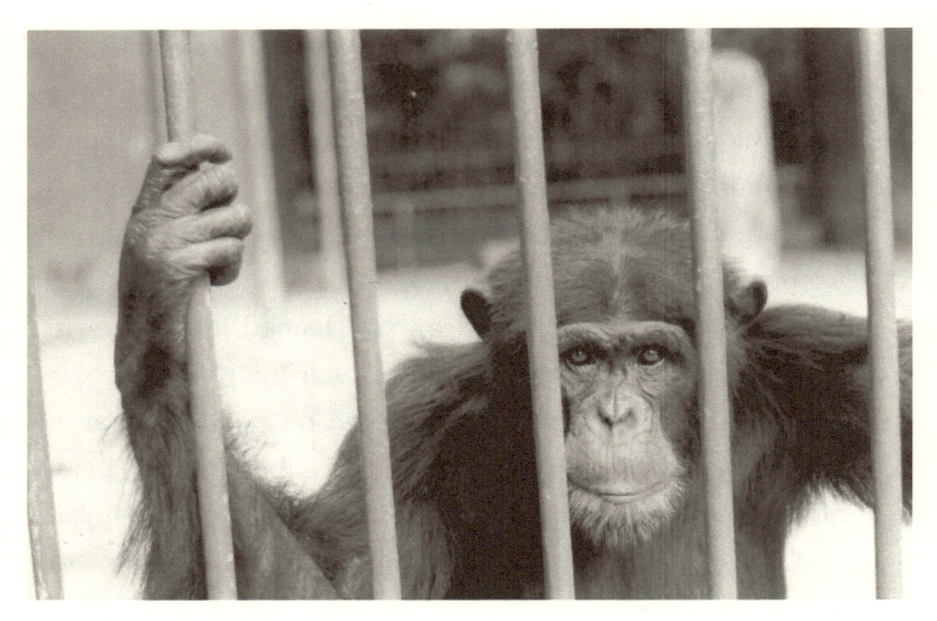

Tali adjusting to prison life.

To my surprise, Tali hesitantly approached the bars, eyes downcast to the floor. He reached out through the bars—slowly this time—and dabbed some of the blood from my face with his index finger. He touched the blood to his own lips, then retreated to the corner with his back to us. His body posture suggested a scolded, sulking child.

By the end of my zoo internship, I had been attacked by more animals than most people can identify.

Back to Africa | 119

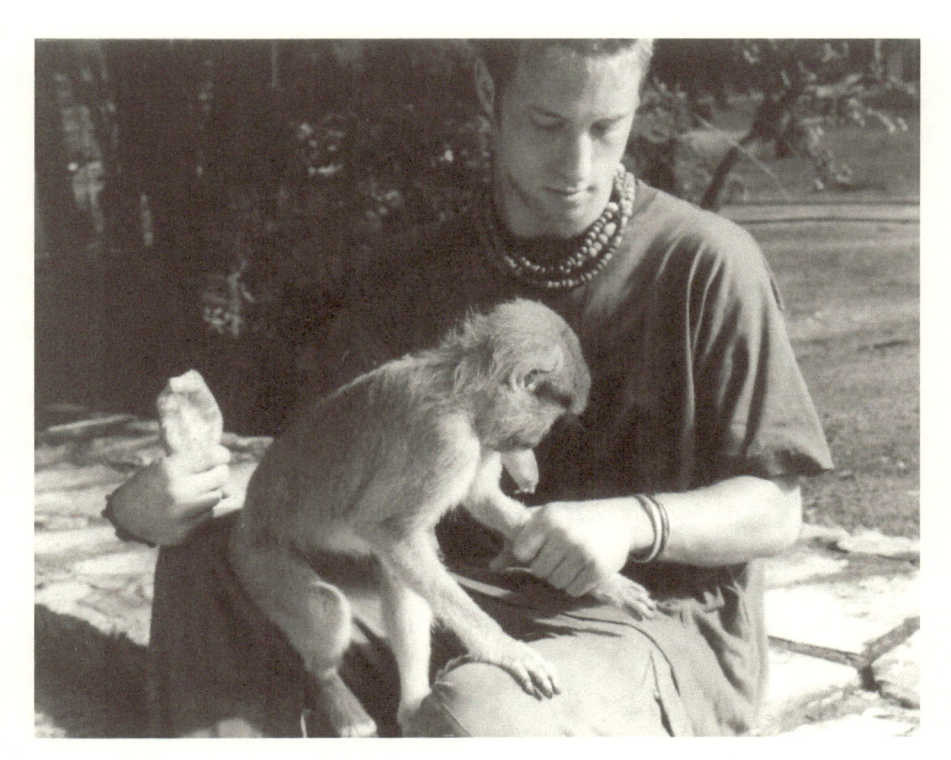

Me and my cousin 618,000th removed (on my mom's side).

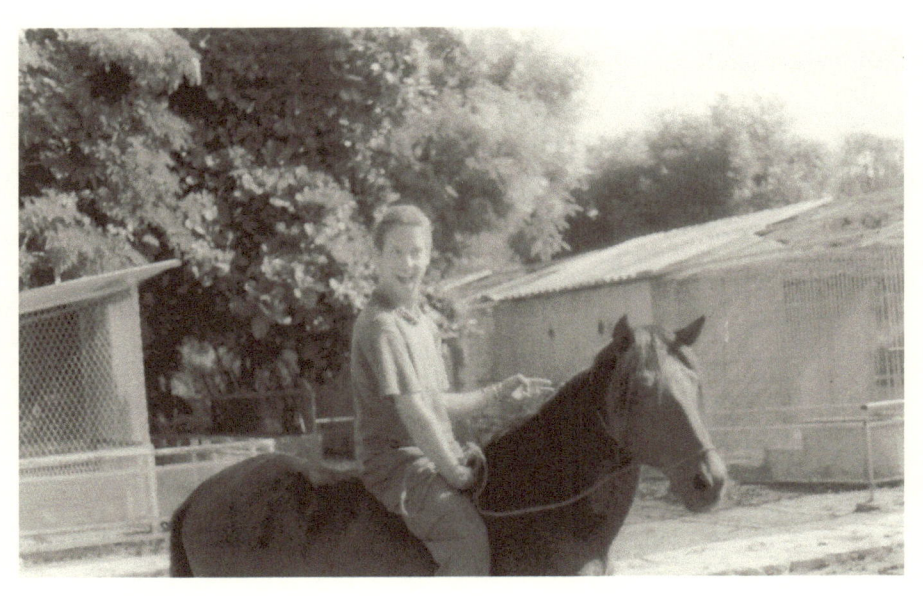

My last time barebacking.

THE BOOBOO MONKEY

"*Amnaa bena idée,*" I said in French and Wolof. *I have an idea.* Usman raised an eyebrow. "I want you to put me on display. I will be your newest attraction at the zoo."

Usman's eyes shined at the thought of it. "This is perfect. I know right where you should go. This is where I always thought you belonged. You are a little *golo*," he said, walking around with a simian strut and making monkey noises.

"*Kofuma!*" I shot back.

"I know you're not joking, and I'm sure you will be our new star attraction. This is a very good prank, and I know the visitors will reward you with many peanuts and maybe even a banana. I will tell the boss you are doing this next Sunday," Usman said, pretending to eat a bug that he'd plucked out of my long hair.

Three days later, the heavy metal bars slid down with a convincing *thunk*. I was barefoot and almost nude, wearing only thin gray shorts. Usman gave me one last skeptical look and a big rectangular smile, before he slipped the padlock into the chain around the bars. I watched through the bars as my new neighbor, a lone silverback gorilla named Paco, ran up and punched the thin, red metal door that was the only thing separating us, easily denting it. I was invading his home; he had two side-by-side cages, and every day he switched from one to the other. The one he wasn't in was cleaned while he dirtied the other one with sour-smelling poop, banana peels, watermelon rinds, potato skins, and cigarette butts.

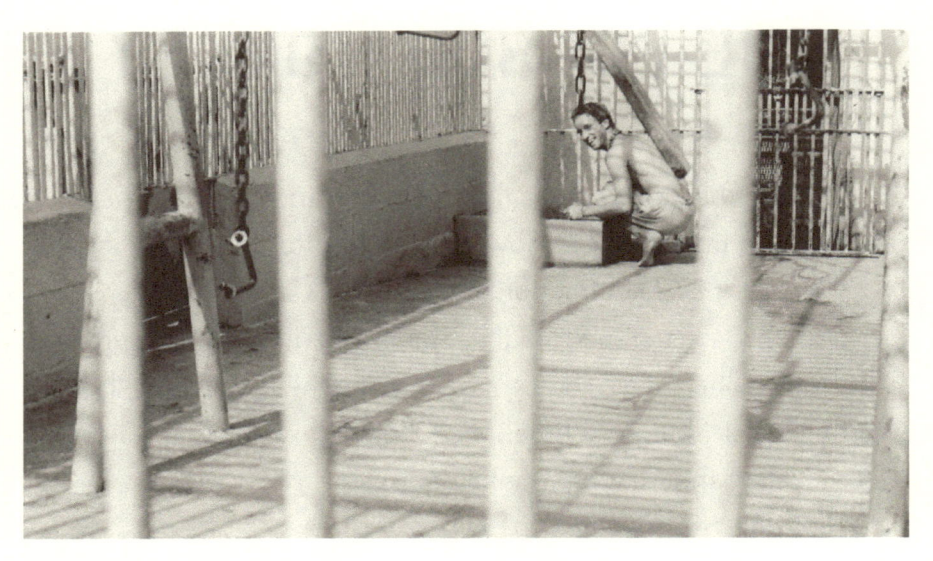

Me at the watering hole.

Paco had come to the zoo with his sister when they were very young, likely orphaned by hunters. His sister had died soon after, leaving Paco alone and starved for affection. The keepers told me stories of how young Paco wouldn't let them leave the cage; he would wrap his strong arms and legs around them and cling to them like a giant koala. Even as a youngster, Paco was soon stronger than any man, even Usman. Once, a keeper had been kept in a friendly hostage situation for four hours. The humans had to resort to spraying Paco with water or poking him with broomsticks to escape his cage.

I had become close to this beast and especially loved his gigantic, craggy, dark-black hands. Under Usman's watchful eye, I had become one of the three people on Earth who could pet him —after learning his favorite snacks and bribing him.

I gave him a respectful wide berth as I tenderly walked across the rough cement floor. Paco watched with his deep-set, piercing eyes as he shaved a potato with his incisors and, with two massive snapping sounds, devoured it. Before this day, our relationship was keeper and animal, but now I was in his cage, a co-captive. I could tell he was curious, but he was also a gorilla, so he was only capable of showing it by smashing stuff—like most male primates.

The punishing African sun created intense shadows through the bars as I explored my cage. There was a broken metal swing hanging by one chain (Paco's handiwork), as well as two well-worn chains hanging from the ceiling that connected in the middle. I had seen Paco swing his muscular bulk on these chains many times. They would now be my only source of entertainment. In the corner was a concrete basin full of water, lined with a thick layer of slimy green algae I had spent the previous two months trying to scrub away.

Usman came around the front of the cage, his dark skin glistening with sweat, his white teeth gleaming with happiness. He yelled at me in Wolof, "Hello monkey!"

"*Ooogh, ooogh,*" I replied.

"If anyone asks, I didn't put you in there," Usman said. And with a wink, he lumbered away in his knee-high rubber boots and Senegalese army fatigues, past the mean leopard, then on past Claws, the big Siberian tiger.

I gave a few ape-like explorations of my cage and crawled into the dark concrete room in the corner that Paco used as his den. It was about ten feet by ten feet, with a surprisingly high ceiling. The den room was filled with freshly laid hay, but still had the pungent odor of a gorilla's bedroom. The concrete walls magnified any noise, and my voice echoed back to me. Earlier, Usman and I had cleaned this room, pulling out old hay soaked with gorilla urine and thousands of dung beetles and roaches. It looked like it hadn't been done in months.

"I always lay fresh hay for the new monkeys to acclimate them," Usman said as he hoisted a big bale through the door.

Paco was a flirt with me, but he played the tough guy when other people were around. We had a game where he'd wrap his arm around his head, bite the inside of his elbow, and make a low growling noise. Then he'd put his other arm on the ground and stick his silvery butt in the air. This meant it was okay to pet him. I'd slide my hand, snake-like, through the bars and smack him on his butt and his big, tight beer belly. He'd grunt and growl with joy.

The second he got out of that posture, I would snap my hand back out of the cage. We could play this game for hours, and often did, but I always wondered what would happen if he got hold of my wrist. Tali had easily bashed me against the bars; Paco could surely rip my arm off like Chewbacca.

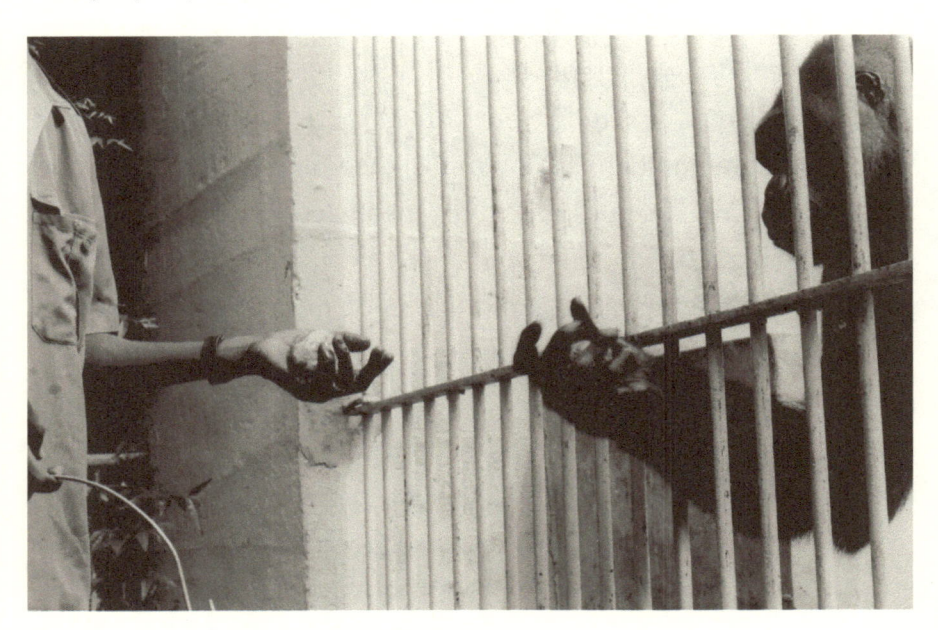

Paco working on his hip handshake.

The zoo was opening in a few minutes. The straw itched, but I rolled in it, anyway. I hoped to attain the same look Paco had most mornings when he came out of his dark room with pieces of hay stuck to his back, like little fishing boats out at sea.

As he ran along the bars, Paco brushed his shoulder against them and shook the whole metal frame of our cage. He wanted me to come out of the back room, his bedroom. I peeked my head out.

"*Ooogh*," I said. His dark eyes studied me, wondering what I was doing in his bedroom, like a big brother might. He stood tall and alert, sniffed hard with his two crater-like nostrils, and wrapped his thick fingers around the bars. I hopped toward him, and he retreated to a far corner. He brushed a pile of potato skins into his hand and hurled them at me.

I heard Usman tromping over an uneven rock path. He hopped over the green barrier fence and handed me a plastic milk container filled with water. "It's going to be hot today," he said, then walked away to open the zoo.

I took a large swig and carried the jug into my hay den, hiding it out of sight. I rolled out and sprang onto the bars, then climbed up and hung from the crossbars. I swung back and forth for a few minutes until I had red calluses and flecks of turquoise paint on my hands. I dropped to the cement floor; my arms burned and my feet hurt from the sharp landing.

A man wearing a long, flowing robe rounded the corner with two children. I scampered back into the cold confines of my lair. My heart fluttered, and my palms were now sweating, stinging the blistering calluses. This was it. No dress rehearsal. No stage director to shove me out there. It was time to perform.

I heard squeaks of joy from the two little girls as they passed the cranky leopard. Paco could smell the salted peanuts they carried, and he eagerly paced back and forth. As they passed my cage, I hid in the shadows, watching. Paco reached one hand through the cage and shook the bars with his other in his well-practiced extortion. It worked. The man threw a plastic bag of peanuts into the bowl of Paco's hand.

Paco pulled the packet through the bars, tore the plastic off with his teeth, and shook the peanuts into his wet mouth. Before he was done chewing, he had his hand out, beckoning for more. The visitors smiled, delighted by his begging. I poked my head out. The only one who noticed was Paco, and I was only competition to him. The squeaks of red colobus and green vervet monkeys stole the attention of the little girls, and they ran off.

Once the attention had moved to the monkeys, I came out of hiding and onto my stage. Paco bit his inner elbow, so I reached through the bars into his cage and gave him a few quick pats. He broke out of his posture, jumped six feet straight up, and slid his hands down the bars. I jumped up and did the same. We went back and forth as if we were on a teeter-totter; as soon as he landed, I popped up. We had never played this game before, and I was fascinated that Paco was just making it up.

Then the game changed. He ran down to the front corner of his cage, and I chased him. As soon as he reached the end, he came tearing back past me, clutching the bars and pulling himself along. When I got to the back of my cage, I waited a few seconds, then rushed to the front of the cage, as he ran back and punched that red metal door, making a huge, echoing *boom*. Back and forth we went until we were both panting. Then the game stopped abruptly.

Paco's dark-marble eyes looked past me, and without turning,

I knew we were being watched. I spun sharply and found a pack of local high school boys gawking at us, smoking. It was too late to hide now. Their mouths and eyes were in a competition to see who could open wider as they took in this unfinished ape. This was a treat they were not expecting.

Paco loped to the front of the cage in hopes of more peanuts, or maybe even a Marlboro. He had picked up the nasty habit of smoking from visitors who came without peanuts and mistook his extended hand to mean, *I need a smoke.* They'd throw one in, and he would pick the lit cigarette up gingerly and take short drags, holding the smoke in for a few seconds before exhaling. Cheers came from the spectators, and all the zookeepers knew Paco was at it again. The zoo obviously frowned on any of the animals smoking, but I felt like the poor guy deserved one. He lived his entire life in a stinky cage; that's what cigarettes are for. If not now, then when?

The best way to get a 450-pound beast to stop smoking is to spray water at him until the cigarette goes out. Paco was remarkable at defending the cherry of his cigarette with his giant umbrella of a hand, shielding it with his body, and sneaking puffs when he could.

I looked from the boys to Paco and grunted twice. Then I hopped to the front of the cage, with my head jerking side to side and my arms out at jaunty angles. My actions were purposeful and ape-like, but what sold them were the involuntary motions from the palsy. The teenage boys saw me as a creature, reminding me of so many cruel tormentors back in the States. I guess teenagers are shitty all over the world. As I approached, smirks turned to frowns, and they all backpedaled. I crouched down and extended a crooked hand, as I had seen my teacher Paco do so many times before. The boys' faces contorted in bewildered horror.

"Ooogh, ooogh."

"What is that?" one of the boys whispered in Wolof.

"I don't know," replied another.

Then they were bombarded by a shower of potato skins hurled by my jealous neighbor who was used to being the center of attention. The kids ran in several directions.

I shook my head and laughed. It reminded me of the time earlier in the summer when I had come around the corner to find a group of teens collecting rocks to throw at Paco. I had surprised them in Wolof. "What are you doing?"

"Nothing," one boy said as he dropped the rocks back into the sand.

"Would you throw those rocks at that gorilla if he wasn't in that cage?"

"We weren't throwing rocks!" defended the spokesman for the group.

"If you throw rocks again, you're going to have to leave," I said, trying to keep my composure. Upon being challenged by a goofy toubab, these boys puffed up their chests and began to spread around me, as if to suggest, *there are more of us than there are of you.* The rocks around us could just as easily be thrown at me. But I had experience with packs of wild dogs from years ago, and I stood my ground, glaring, letting them know I wasn't messing around. It was a Mexican standoff in Africa. Just like after Fatou had attacked me, there was a palpable stillness to the zoo, and I knew the animals were watching.

Breaking the tension, Paco stood on his hind legs and rushed forward, pounding his hands against his rock-hard chest, making a rapid *paco paco paco* drum-like sound. Then he crashed his

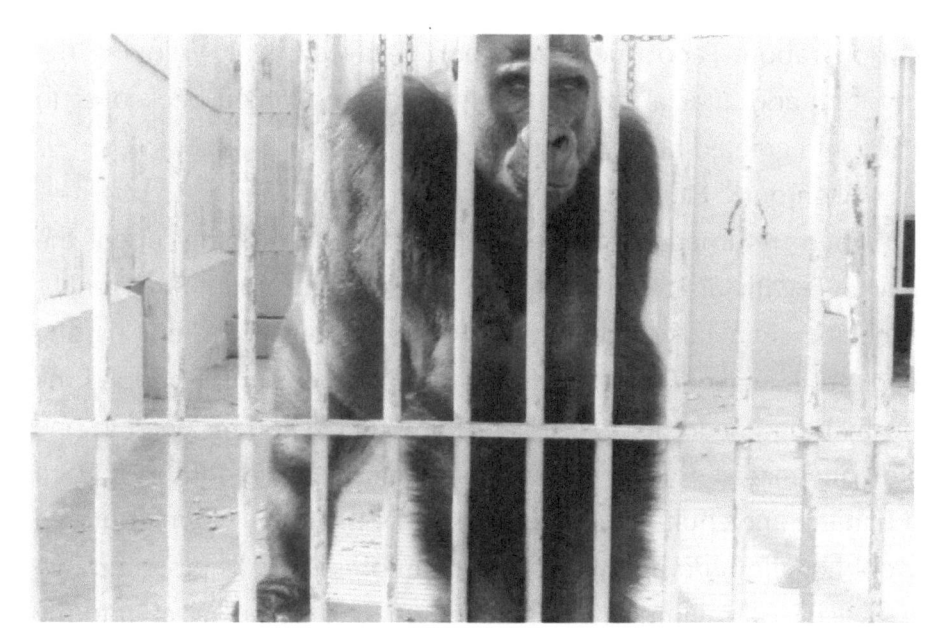

POV: You're locked in a cage next to a silverback gorilla.

shoulder into the bar. *Thounggg.* The kids scattered in every direction, even through hedges. All the hair on my body stood up, and I got goosebumps. "Thanks," I said, but Paco wouldn't look at me. Just like with my palsy punch, Paco had caught those bullies off guard. *Game recognize game.*

A cloud covered the sun as a new visitor approached Paco and me. I tucked back into my den and pushed my head out to join Paco in sizing up a short, wrinkly man, with thinning white hair and round glasses. He approached Paco's side of the cage. I watched from my cool confines as Paco held his hand out for peanuts, clearly recognizing this fellow. The old man must have caught a glimpse of motion in my den and tried to pick me out of the shadows. I grunted loudly and threw out hay. The little man gently took off his glasses and cleaned them. He was clearly curious about Paco's new neighbor. I stayed silent, enjoying the mystery, and after a few moments, the man walked back over to Paco and greeted him with an air of familiarity.

"Bonjour!" He tossed Paco a packet of nuts.

Paco returned the greeting by expertly ripping open the package with his teeth and gulping down the treat. The French-speaking man talked quietly to Paco, but his eyes kept darting back to my cage. Enough was enough. With a grunt, I popped my bushy blond head out of the den. The man cocked his head to one side and stared at me with astonishment. He absently threw Paco a banana and shuffled toward my side of the cage. I came out in a wobbly gallop, doing my best gorilla impression. I climbed up two bars using all my limbs, slid back down, and dashed back into my den. It was a display I had seen Paco do many times. The man rubbed the sweat from his brow with his forearm, blinked twice so hard I could hear it, and then tore off for the zoo entrance as fast as his little old legs could carry him. I sat and chuckled as Paco looked at me sideways as if to say, "Hey man, I was working here!"

Usman returned along the same path, his square shoulders bouncing with laughter.

"What did you say to that old man?" he asked.

I shrugged and gave him my classic crooked smile.

"He wanted to know what species of animal you are, and where we got you," Usman said. I found this hard to believe, but he continued, "I told him that you are what they call a booboo monkey from the mountains of Congo." He could barely get the words out around his laughter. "He just ran out the front gate when I told him that." Usman clapped his hands to show how quickly the man had left.

I grinned and said in a low growl, "Booboo."

Usman walked off to tend to other animals, wiping tears of laughter from his eyes.

Ten minutes later, the man was back with a bigger bag of goodies. I was sitting with my legs hanging out of the bars, my arms flexing and twitching. His sweet, old face had a look that mixed bewilderment, horror, and curiosity. I shoved my left hand toward him while my right hand curled around the hot bars. He looked from me to the peanuts in his hand, and I grunted loudly. He threw them to me, but they fell short, landing in the sand before my cage. I knew there was no way he was jumping over the safety barrier to get them for me.

"*Ooogh, ooogh,*" I said, pretending to be upset.

Paco judged all of this silently: He would never miss a bag of peanuts.

The man hesitated, then reached into his goodie bag and pulled out more salty peanuts. He held them up in front of my face and said in French, more to himself than to me, "Are you ready this time?"

He threw the bag of nuts in a high, slow arc, and I snapped them through the bars. Just like Paco, I peeled the plastic off with my teeth and emptied the contents into my mouth. The old man smiled shyly, shook his head, and walked toward Paco, who was growing more and more impatient. He threw the gorilla a few more packs, and I grunted with jealousy.

Shortly after this, the old man walked away to finish his loop of the zoo, still pondering the mystery of the booboo monkey. To this day I'll never know if that man was in on the joke, or if he died thinking he saw the rarest of all primates.

Usman came by, pushing a wheelbarrow brimming with a

medley of animal shit. "It's midday," he said. It was time for siesta. "We're gonna close the zoo now until three. Would you like to come out to eat lunch like a human?"

I shook my head no; my host brothers would be bringing me food soon and, perhaps more importantly, I didn't want to break character. Sure enough, Papis, Malik, and Sheikh came flapping up in their flip-flops, carrying a big bowl of rice and meat. They started to laugh uncontrollably.

"Bamba, how are you?" Papis asked.

Before I could even make a grunt, Usman said, "That's Booboo, not Bamba."

My brothers laughed, not sure what to make of the whole situation. Usman jumped the fence, and Papis handed him the bowl and a spoon.

"Stay Back! Don't try to escape!" Usman yelled theatrically as he unlocked the door and slid the bowl in. I ran forward. Usman slammed the cage door back down just in time. I grabbed the bowl and ran back into the comforts of my den. I could hear them giggling. My brothers asked me to come out, and I threw the spoon through the bars into the sand. They laughed even harder, loving the performance.

"The booboo monkey doesn't know what a spoon is for," Usman said, retrieving it and handing it back to the boys.

"We'll be back after siesta," my brothers called to me, leaving with smiles from ear to ear.

Usman stayed a few minutes longer and talked at me like the animal I now was. "I'm going to go eat lunch. Don't pinch yourself on the chain," he said.

I knew that he never brought lunch to eat. He would lie on a reed mat in front of the zoo, in the shade of an acacia tree, with all the other zookeepers.

Paco and I now had three hours to get to know each other even better. I sat in my cool room on a bale of hay, eating rice and goat meat. My host mother had prepared a special meal. I wasn't used to eating meat during the day, and she had treated me with all the choicest morsels, like trachea. At least that's what I think it was. It chewed like a meat-flavored piece of bubble gum.

I could hear Paco next door, shuffling back and forth, curiously sniffing the air. Then I heard the unnerving sound of bending metal. I swallowed hard and poked my head out to see Paco's black banana fingers wrapped around the red metal door, pulling it open to see what the new smell might be.

"That's it. That's the end of me," I told myself. "Siesta is gonna finish, and they're gonna find their new booboo monkey in pieces all over his cage." I could scream for Usman; maybe he wasn't out of earshot yet. He'd for sure hear my screams when Paco twisted my head off like the cap on a soda.

I remembered the stories of Paco when he was young, and how he had craved companionship—perhaps he would just keep me like a pet, like Koko with her kitten. I shuddered at the image of Paco carrying me like a newborn, force-feeding me a yam and a cigarette. I crawled out of my hiding spot and approached the door—better to confront him than just wait for him to burst in.

Thank God he just wanted to play.

Paco let go, jumped up, and slid down the bars excitedly. After a little time playing our usual game—to ease my terror of being dismembered—I relaxed. I had the big bowl of rice and goat bits, and knew I couldn't eat it all myself, so I crawled back into my den and brought it out. Paco's eyes widened, and he sniffed real hard, trying to get an angle to see what was in the bowl. I scooped out a handful and threw it into his massive mitt. Greasy rice and meat weren't part of his usual diet, but this might be a matter of life or death for me, and I knew Paco loved food. We sat together, handful for me, handful for him, back and forth, until the bowl was empty. I had seen Paco eat a lot of treats, and this was clearly an all-timer for him. He had been a strict vegan his entire life, and I felt a pang of regret for breaking his streak.

I carried the empty bowl into the den area, got my water bottle, and came back out. Paco was already slurping from his concrete basin, but when he saw the water bottle, he stopped and came over to me. He poked his lips through the bars, and I put the bottle up to them; I'd seen this done before. His prehensile lips wrapped around it like fingers, and he took half the bottle down in one gulp. My belly was full, but I didn't think Paco's beer belly could ever be full. I'd seen him eat two watermelons, three cucumbers, eight potatoes, and four apples in one sitting, then wash it all down with a cigarette.

I convinced him that I had no more food, and he initiated play —back and forth, up and down. In the corner of his cage, he shimmied up the bars, got to the top, flipped upside down, and grabbed on with his hind legs. I had never seen him do this before. He held this position effortlessly for a good ten minutes. I reached in, slapped his belly like a beach ball, and grabbed his arm and burnt bratwurst fingers. Then, for the first time, I petted his face, scratched under his chin, tickled his ears, and caressed his eyebrows. His nose and mouth had no fur on them and felt like an old person's skin, soft and worn. He loved it. He leaned his neck into me and laughed with little chuffs and twinkling eyes. I had never seen even Usman dare to touch Paco's face; our friendship had crossed an amazing threshold. It took absolute trust to put my fingers anywhere near this Goliath's mouth, with its 1,300 psi of biting force; my fingers would just be baby carrots to him.

Two hours passed. I was sweating profusely and retreated back to my den, out of the blazing sun. The empty bowl of rice was covered with ants. Embracing my new animal life, I scooped some writhing rice and popped it into my mouth. They were sour and a little crunchy. The original Sour Patch Kids. I took a piss in the corner, then sat with my back against the cool concrete wall and watched dust particles settle against my sweaty skin. The shadows were different now, falling toward the front of the cage. Paco was silent for some time, perhaps contemplating if I was going to live next to him forever.

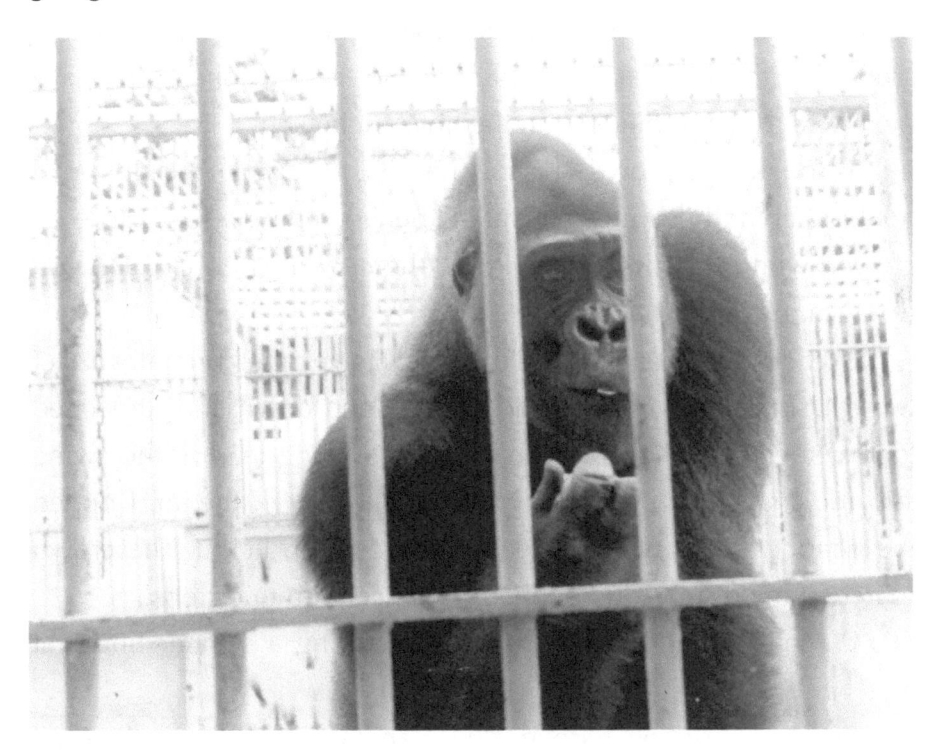

Paco studying his new roommate.

The zoo reopened, and customers trickled back in. Emboldened by my time in the cage and the bonding with Paco, I fully stepped into my role as the booboo monkey, freshly acquired from the mountains of Congo. Faces gathered around my cage and watched me. First five people, then ten, then too many to count. There were shouts in Wolof and French, inquiries and debates about what I could possibly be. More peanuts and fruit were thrown, encouraging me to perform. I threw half the fruit and snacks I got to Paco, who greedily devoured them. He didn't do the same for me; he was clearly the alpha of this operation.

People baited me, "We know you can understand us!"

Others chimed in playfully, "You're crazy, that's a monkey."

Pretty women flirtatiously taunted me, and I tried to ignore them despite being a hormone-driven monkey. I occasionally grunted with pleasure. If people had no food to offer, all I gave them was a cold shoulder—in the hot African sun.

Through the crowd, I saw the top of Usman's bald head bobbing up and down as he walked between the hedges. His eyes glowed with joy as he shouted over the crowd, "Booboo! Do you want some candy, Booboo?"

I reacted the same way I'd seen all the other primates react when Usman was around. I hopped up and down and screeched loudly, then climbed up the bars, took a flying leap at the swing set, and snagged a perfectly thrown sucker out of the air. I ripped the wrapper away with my teeth and began to lick it. The crowd roared at my display and peppered Usman with questions.

"What is that?" one man asked, pointing a slender finger at me.

"That's a booboo monkey," Usman said as he turned to me and gave a little wink. "Booboo!"

"*Eeeiii!*" I said, then pretended to pick a bug out of my hair and eat it.

Usman put up a folding chair just far enough away that he didn't seem suspicious, watching the spectacle and having a good laugh.

My host brothers showed up again, nudging their way to the front. I grunted to acknowledge them. More people filtered in; the word was out about the zoo's newest oddity. Some people fed Paco fruits and vegetables, and for the most part he was calm, except for the occasional shotgunning of potato peels and wet peanut shells into the crowd.

Now, questions were directed at me personally. "Booboo, are you French? American? German?"

No response from me, except picking up stray peanuts and fidgeting with my blond leg hairs. There was one especially beautiful woman in the front who didn't speak French or Wolof, only English. She was asking me everything, trying to get me to break. She even asked me to marry her. I grunted loudly. I nonchalantly flexed my biceps and tried to make my six-pack into an eight-pack. For fifteen minutes, she tried everything, flirting with me, teasing me, escalating into some R-rated questions about my anatomy below the belt.

Out of frustration, she yelled, "You're crazy!" This was one of the only English words everyone in the audience knew. People laughed.

I gave a low growl in Wolof. "*Yaa ma gëna dof.*"

The crowd laughed even harder and nudged each other. "I told you he could talk!"

The woman frowned. "What did he say? What did he say?"

A tall British student in the back piped up, "He said you're crazier than him!"

I clambered back into my concrete bunker, hoping the echoes of my own laughter wouldn't carry out. After a moment, I jumped back into character and heeded the beckoning calls from my fans. I threw my water bottle like a playful primate, followed it, and took a few monkey sips to wash down all the salty peanuts.

I brought it over to Paco and put it to his eager lips. Shouts of astonishment and disgust rang through the crowd. Encouraged by their engagement, I put the bottle back to my lips and was met with a roar of absolute revulsion. I saw my Ndiaye brothers whispering, and I knew I'd have some explaining to do to my host mother.

The crowd thinned. So much for my new fans. I looked over to where Usman sat and saw him talking to a man with his wife and two young children. He pointed over to my cage, and my adrenaline spiked to a new level as I recognized the man. He was the doctor who I had visited three weeks earlier for malaria.

I remembered the doctor's engaging bedside manner. He was funny, and he spoke English. He was curious about my adventures at the zoo, so I had invited him to visit, but why today of all days? He thanked Usman and walked toward me, concern growing on his face. I had already been an oddity back in his office—a White man with cerebral palsy—but this was a whole new level.

I squatted on my haunches. Fluent in all three languages, he tentatively tried greeting me in Wolof, then French, then resorted to English, all to no avail.

Instead, I greeted him with my best primate grunts. He nervously laughed, and his children shifted, hiding behind his legs, each one peeking a light-brown eye at me. His wife wasn't sure how to look at me, so I teased her by grunting suggestively.

"Do you remember who I am?" the doctor asked, hesitant and hopeful.

I stood up, extended one finger, and poked it to the top of my left buttcheek where he had given me the shot for malaria. He chuckled with relief as he ushered his children further away from the cage.

"I understand," he said, but he didn't look convinced that I hadn't gone bananas. The fish eagles chirped loudly, as he gently shook his head and walked away.

I tried to pick up a peanut with my toes and let my adrenaline cool. A fresh crowd formed to watch me, and another familiar face showed up.

It was Kamera, with off-white chipped teeth and his face like wax melting to the ground. He was the man at the zoo who trimmed the hedges and kept them symmetrical. I never thought he liked me much after he chased me around with his rusty hedge clippers, because I had taken his picture without asking. All that aside, he was now standing in front of me in civilian clothes.

"What is that?" he asked the man next to him through the gap in his teeth.

The man puffed up his chest and said, "That's a booboo monkey."

Kamera smiled. *"Ah bon?"*

"Yes, he comes from the mountains of Congo."

"Oh, really? Does he sleep in there?"

"Oh, yes." The man went on in Wolof. "They caught him a few years ago."

"Really?"

I tried not to look at Kamera to prevent us both from laughing. I had to get up and retreat into my den. When I came back out,

Kamera had left, but I saw him laughing with Usman. The legend of the booboo monkey was growing.

The other man was still in front of my cage with about twenty other people, playing the role of the foremost expert on me. Paco swatted the water from his basin, spraying the crowd and me with liquid that smelled like gorilla poop and algae. He ran to the back of his cage and punched a metal wall. It sounded like thunder rolling over us.

"Is that your brother?" a woman yelled out as she pointed to Paco.

"Yes, it's the white monkey," someone else shouted.

My host brothers jumped the barrier in front of my cage to collect all the peanuts that had fallen short. The youngest, Malik, grew brave and careless. Just as I had seen Tali do to me, I snatched his wrist, yanked his arm in, and started licking and biting him gently. Malik shrieked, and Papis and Sheikh grabbed his legs in a human tug-of-war. Everyone started yelling and screaming.

Usman marched over with the legitimate authority of a veteran zookeeper. He used his tone that was reserved for Earth's apex predators. "Booboo, drop it!"

I let go, and Papis and Sheikh fell back in the sand, with Malik landing on top of them.

"Okay," Usman said, "enough is enough. Time to get out of there."

I shrieked. This time, I really was disappointed. I felt I had finally come into my role as a captive primate. Usman unlocked the padlock and unwrapped the chain. Sensing my departure, Paco rammed the metal door with his fist, and the crowd collectively jumped. Usman strained to lift the heavy cage door, and the audience in front began to brace themselves while brave children came closer to the door, making sure they had a wide escape route behind them.

Usman crawled into the small cage opening, and I pounced on his back. "Enough, enough," he said.

I stopped, collected my belongings from my den, put on my shirt, and crawled back out into the five o'clock sun. I looked into my audience.

"*Merci beaucoup,*" I said. I waved to Paco, who wouldn't look at me. He was unhappy that I was leaving and would be mad at me for a while. We had bonded, but more importantly, I had brought a surplus of extra goodies his way.

On the way out of the cage, I had skinned my knee. As I shakily jumped the green barrier fence, people gave me an oh-so-wide berth and observed me with a mix of curiosity and raw terror. The veil between my primate life and the real world had been lifted, and it felt strange to walk out among the humans. I headed toward the entryway, passing the Siberian tiger. He purred at me to pet him, but I didn't stop. The woman who offered to marry me was hiding behind her friends, and I winked at her. I reached the entrance of the zoo and saw a white face, strangely familiar.

"You must be Joshua," the woman said and introduced herself as Molly.

I recognized her as a scholarly friend of my father's whom I had been instructed to find two months ago and totally didn't do. Molly had done endless work with women's movements in Senegal and was one of the world's best non-native Wolof speakers.

"What did you do today?" she asked in English almost

accusingly, noticing I was trailing a parade of gawking onlookers.

I still shook with adrenaline and grunted at her. "I had my friends here lock me in a cage next to the gorilla," I said, half in English and half in Wolof.

"Why on Earth would you do that?"

"I figured everyone is always staring at me, anyway. Might as well give them something to stare at."

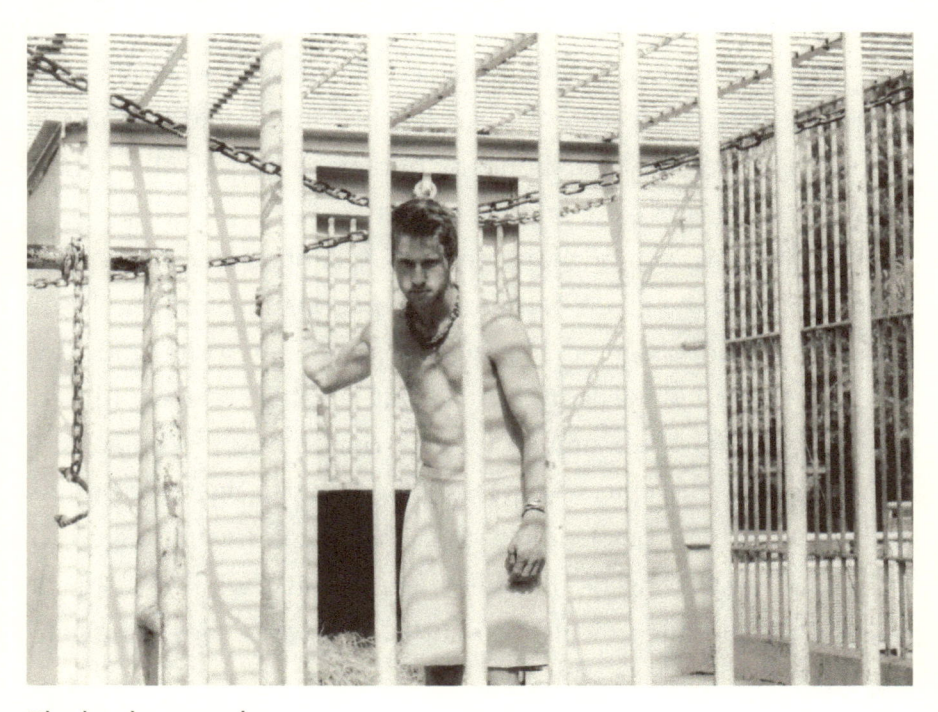

The booboo monkey.

THOR IN THE WOODS

When I was in college at Evergreen, I spent most of my time wandering through the rainforest that made up the thousand acres of campus. Before I moved to Olympia, everyone warned me that Washington was always dreary and gray, and that it was the suicide capital of the world. I told myself I would go outside every day, sunny or not, to stay above ground.

The campus was nestled in the rainforest, and my friends and I built an elaborate fort from salvaged tarps, ropes, and boards. It was my favorite place to study. I listened to my textbooks on tape and cooked Top Ramen over a fire. That's where I perfected my fire-building skills, working with that perpetually wet wood.

I went out late at night and picked my way through the drenched underbrush without a flashlight, a skill I learned at Camp Sunrise. I am somehow more graceful when I am navigating through the woods. My unpredictable nature on a flat surface can knock me on my ass, but outside, the uneven earth will move up to meet my feet. It's my controlled chaos. I will say, the one thing I learned was to always wear shoes.

Once, when I was eleven years old, I was visiting my oldest friend Nick at his family's cabin, running through the Wisconsin woods, barefoot as usual. I ran behind the shed and immediately stepped my right foot down on a rusty nail. It stabbed deep into my flesh. I howled and hopped around. Struggling to keep my balance, a new and greater pain shot into my left foot. I fell to my back, both feet sticking straight up, with a decaying board attached to my right foot and two porcupine quills lodged in the left. I started laughing. *Oh, it's gonna be this kind of life, huh?*

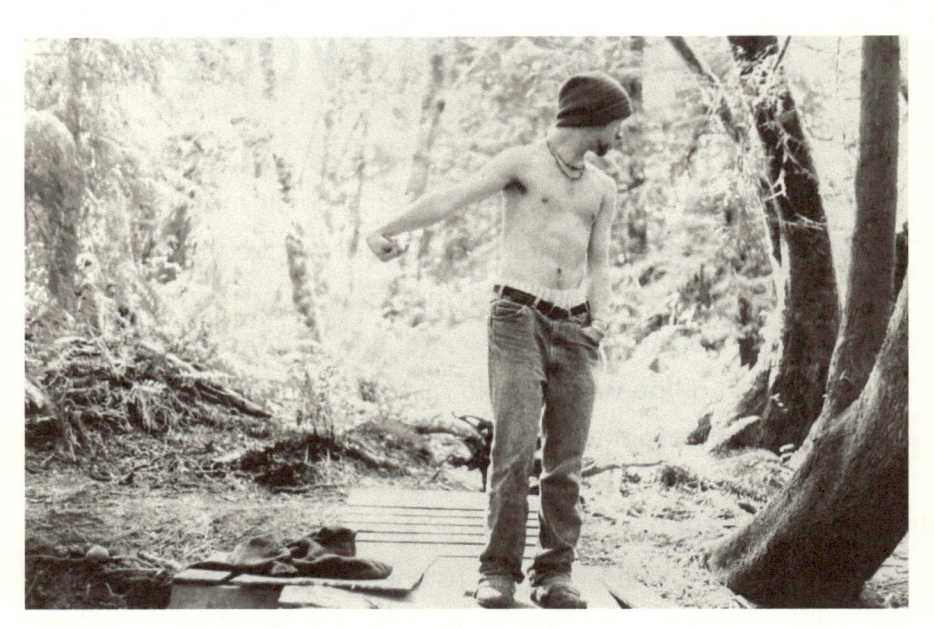

Going through my boy band phase.

Early in my freshman year, I was on one of my nighttime adventures in the woods when I ran into an older guy roaming around in the dark without a flashlight. After that we kept passing each other, night after night, until we finally had to address it.

"So what are you doing out here?" he asked, with a voice raspy enough to scrape paint off brick.

"I was wondering the same thing about you, man."

He looked to be in his fifties, a sharp-featured, lanky guy, with a five o'clock shadow and an Adam's apple like a knot on a tree. His wavy blond hair was cut short and going on gray. The first night we met, as on most nights thereafter, he was wearing a dress shirt tucked into his khaki shorts with tube socks pulled up to his knees and scuzzy brown loafers. He had three tallboys hanging by a plastic ring in one hand, and the other hand kept fidgeting with his menthol cigarette. He looked glaringly out of place in the woods, but moved through them as if he belonged there. Just like me.

"My name's Thor," he said casually, as if it wasn't the name of a god. He quickly added, "I've got a rowboat down there." He gestured with the glowing tip of his cigarette toward the Puget Sound. "Want to go out and look at the stars?"

"Okay. You're not going to kill me or molest me or anything, are you?"

"Not unless you give me good reason," he said over his shoulder as he disappeared down the hill into the darkness.

I followed him, wondering what would be a good reason to molest me, until we reached the spot where the forest abruptly met the beach. Thor burrowed into a mean, thorny bush and emerged with a pair of beat-up oars. We picked our way down the shore full of jagged, slimy rocks. Thor's boat was overturned among the rocks, a long way from the spot where he hid the oars.

I let him do the rowing. If I'd done it, we'd still be going in circles. Each time he dipped an oar in the water, it excited the fascinating bioluminescent algae, and a trail of bright green light followed us. In the light of the algae, frightened fish rocketed away, leaving a trail behind them like a comet. I pulled out a J and sparked it, then offered it to Thor.

"I don't do drugs," he told me proudly, as he let go of one of the oars to grab the tallboy clutched between his knees.

He rowed us out to a floating 8-by-12-foot, anchored dock, somewhere in the Puget Sound. I got drunk on his shitty beer and stared up at the endless sky. Thor and I were clearly cut from the same cloth. We repeated this ritual often over the next four years, without planning it once.

If I ever learned Thor's last name, I can't remember it now. His house butted up against the Evergreen campus woods, which was why he was always traipsing around in them. He told me he was in politics but never went into any more detail than that. He gave me a test tube full of gold he had panned out of a river, with the same air that he'd hand me a piece of white bread and insist I feed it to one of his ravenous raccoons that visited him daily. To this day, I believe Thor is the Easter Bunny. Let me explain.

One night, toward the end of my senior year, I got the urge to spend a night outside in the woods, like I so often had over the last four years. I was more comfortable sleeping in the dirt than my own bed, so I set off from my apartment at one in the morning, with my tarp, sleeping bag, and trusty machete, all gathered by the door from regular use. I bushwhacked in the dark through a part of the forest I had not yet explored, then threw the tarp down, unrolled my sleeping bag, and promptly fell asleep in the cold, wet air.

I slept soundly until daybreak, when I awoke to the piercing alarm call of a cedar waxwing. A gray fog hung over me in the crisp air, not quite touching my face, stopping a foot or so above the leafy ground. I sat up, still in my sleeping bag, and my right arm struggled to unzip it. I realized that by sitting up, I was now above this strange fog. It was only a six-inch layer, spreading as far as I could see, around the fat ankles of the conifer trees. The short, violent battle between my sleeping bag and me had pushed the fog away enough for me to notice the Easter basket about a foot away from where my head had been.

I say basket, but it was actually clear, plastic Tupperware, big enough to store half a ham. Alas, there was no ham in this basket. It was brimming with plastic, green grass, chocolate-cream eggs, yellow marshmallow chicks, jelly beans, and a handwoven bracelet with JAMAICA sewn into it. It wasn't until I saw the basket that I remembered it was Easter Sunday. I broke out in goosebumps, and not from the chilly fog I was sitting in.

Somebody had visited me in the night. I had written the Easter Bunny off years before, but I couldn't think of any human who would have been able to get this close to me without waking me up, or who would even go to this much trouble just to give me candy. I'd always been a light sleeper—thanks to those Senegalese cockroaches. I hadn't told anyone I was coming out here. I wondered if this basket was intended specifically for me, or if someone happened to be roaming the woods last night, giving out candy, which was even more disturbing. The only person I could imagine doing this was Thor, but I was in a part of the woods that neither of us had ever explored.

When I grilled him later, Thor adamantly denied having anything to do with the basket and asked a few questions for plausible deniability. Later that week, I wrote an article in the school paper asking the responsible party to step forward. I never got a confession.

After watching the VHS tapes of comedians with disabilities in Linda Pickering's office, I was reinvigorated to cannonball back into stand-up. For my last four credits at Evergreen, I designed a course to study motivational speaking and stand-up comedy. Now, I know what you're thinking, and no, it wasn't just renting Richard Pryor tapes and getting high—although that was definitely a major part of it. Studying the greats was more than being blown away by their performance; it was watching their body posture, timing, pauses, and writing, all the way down to the subtle arch of an eyebrow.

My curriculum included writing and performing my own weekly comedy show somewhere in the sleepy little town of

Olympia, which didn't have any comedy venues. At the end of the quarter, my finale would be an hour-long performance on campus.

I found a venue at a local coffee shop and was invited to do ten minutes between two bands. My debut week, all my friends came to support me, and then promptly left before the headlining band finished their soundcheck. The second week, the same thing happened, except there were even more of my people in the audience. The owner of the shop approached me.

"Very funny! Looks like you need your own night." She offered me a full hour on Wednesday nights, and I eagerly accepted.

I started performing an hour of new material every week at that coffee shop. When I say material, know that it was just me awkwardly sitting at a table, telling funny stories, and ad-libbing jokes into them. I called it The Josh Blue Hour. Looking back, with decades of stand-up experience and six recorded hours under my belt, I couldn't possibly do that again. When you watch a professional comedian performing an hour of material, know that it took years to craft.

If I watched The Josh Blue Hour now, I would cringe myself in half, but luckily for me, these were my friends and peers who were there to support me and had no real frame of reference for entry-level stand-up. My energy and enthusiasm made up for my flimsy material, and it kept the audiences engaged and laughing at all the right parts. By the end of the quarter, it was standing room only. I told my roommate Togashi that I felt like a little campfire in the middle of a forest, and my goal after graduating was to spread the fire to as much of the woods as possible.

"If anyone can make a big fire, it's you," Togashi said with fear and admiration. "I've seen it, man."

Performing at the local coffee shop every week was fun, but I had the itch to perform at an actual comedy club and see what a real stand-up stage felt like. So I found the nearest club, up the road in Tacoma, and convinced some friends to drive me to their open-mic night. As the new guy, I was given two minutes of stage time at the top of the show. I had been doing a meandering hour every week, and now I would have to figure out how to be funny in an impossibly small window of time.

The green room was packed with aspiring comics who had their obvious cliques and I was the new rube, fresh out of the woods of Olympia. The host of the show was a cop, and after pointedly ignoring me, he begrudgingly asked for my intro as he pounded toward the stage. Not prepared for this question, I stammered out my name and a generic intro.

The cop-comic proceeded to do the worst ten minutes of comedy I had seen to date, which actually calmed my sizzling nerves. His material was simply stories of blatant police brutality told in the cadence of stand-up. When it was time to bring me up, he further killed the show's non-existent momentum with a hand-wringing, condescending intro about how I was his very special friend.

I walked out and took the mic. "I don't know that motherfucker."

The crowd broke open. I don't remember anything else about that blur of a set; I abandoned the jokes I had mentally prepped and went with the energy of the room. I got consistent laughs, but nothing like my off-the-cuff opening line. I came offstage buzzing with energy, wishing I had more time and a stronger closer. That shit was addictive—my first stand-up set in a real comedy club, in front of people who paid to be there. It was a tiny taste of what was possible.

My college career was coming to a close, and it was time for my grand finale before they released me into the world. I made posters with a silverback gorilla that reminded me of Paco, sticking his tongue out and beneath that, in big letters: IT'S NOT THE PALSY. IT'S THE POT.

Linda helped me secure one of the bigger classrooms for a venue, and we set up the chairs like a proper comedy club. There was no stage and only the fluorescent room lights overhead. On the day of the show, I was delighted and honored to see a slew of faculty members from the past four years. My professors from writing, botany, art, and photography were all there, in addition to my fellow students and scribes; even Thor came out. They all showed up to support me; that gives me goosebumps to this day. They had a genuine interest in what I was doing.

My old botany professor asked, "It's not the palsy, it's the pot?"

"Well..."

"I'm pretty sure we all knew that," she replied.

More than one professor told me that when they saw the posters, everything made sense. I don't remember the material from that show, but I filled the hour. What I do remember is the physical bit I closed with.

"Don't worry about me, folks. I'm going off into the world, and just know that any time I get myself into a sticky predicament, I'm just going to do this..." Then I stood there awkwardly for a beat before jumping straight up into the air. At the pinnacle of my jump, I turned my body sideways, stiff as a board, then dropped hard onto the thin, dingy carpet. It was quite the fall; I used to be

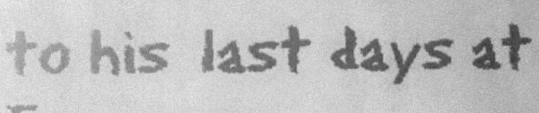

IT'S NOT THE PALSY IT'S THE POT

Josh Blue's comedic tribute to his last days at Evergreen.

See him while you can!

May 30th @ 3pm in Library 1600

Free Munchies!

able to jump freakishly high. The crowd gasped, because no one expects someone with palsy to be able to 1) jump that high, and 2) fall down on purpose.

I don't know how I got away with that as a closer, but the crowd erupted in applause. When I came offstage, people clapped and hugged and high-fived me. As questionable as my comedy may have been, I succeeded in the goals I set for myself, and I got the credits to graduate. My plan was to keep that momentum going and become a big comedy star.

Togashi and I had a barbecue at our apartment to celebrate our impending graduation and invited the student friends we had collected over our four years at Evergreen. I built a fire worthy of Togashi's admiration in the Weber, with sticks and logs that I had dragged out of the woods. It was a small gathering, twenty people at most, but it was a big party. Lots of booze, pot, and mushrooms.

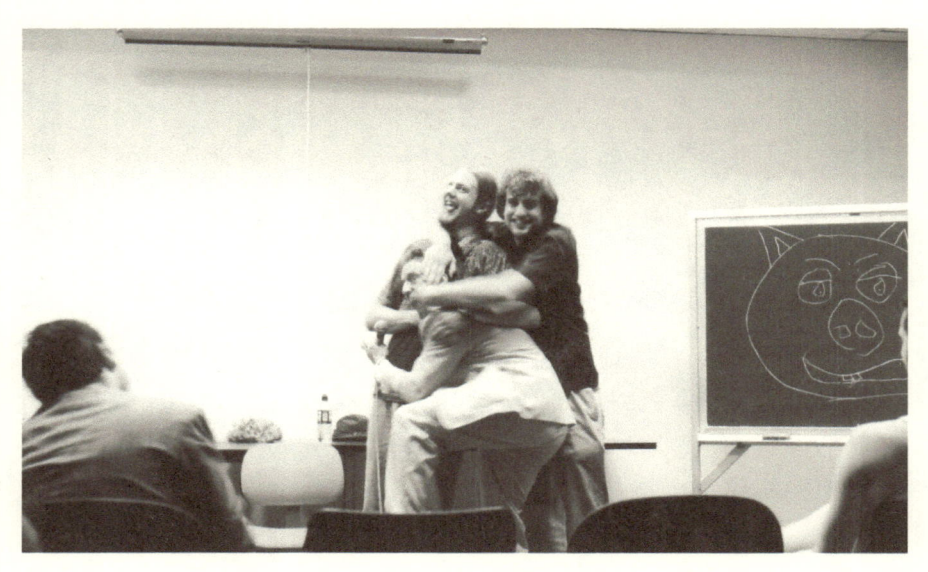

Me, Hal, and our friend Cy celebrating my final comedy performance at Evergreen in front of one of my signature pigs.

My friend Jenny said that the new episode of South Park was airing that night. She suggested we watch the show before we ate the mushrooms. We all piled into the living room in front of our little, 9-inch screen. I'd always been more of a woods guy than a TV guy, but I had seen a few episodes of South Park and knew it was cutting-edge funny. Little did I know just how cutting it was.

One of the first images from the show that night was of wheelchair-bound Timmy tied down in the back of a pickup truck on the way to a scout meeting. Timmy plays to every stereotype of disability: unintelligible, drooling, and wetting himself.

In this episode, Jimmy, a new student with a disability (most likely palsy), fancies himself a comedian and motivational speaker. His first joke was, "I just flew in, and boy, are my crutches tired." It got an awkward laugh, but I could feel my friends' eyes flicking to me to see my reaction. The entire episode was centered on making fun of comedians with disabilities, culminating in a cripple fight at the end. I had been riding high on my comedy aspirations, and now they were being dragged in front of me and slaughtered for the world's amusement.

The longer the episode went on, the bolder my friends' laughs grew, as did their remarks. The closer the friend, the more comfortable he or she was with openly mocking me.

Hal, my best friend and harshest critic, turned to me and asked, "Hey Blue, did you write this?"

"Fuck you, Hal."

"They're stealing your jokes."

"Dick."

"You know what, Joshua," Jenny said. "They pegged you pretty good."

I felt like I had been sucker punched in the stomach; these

were people who had been loyally attending my shows and supporting me. One of the world's biggest comedy shows was skewering my fledgling comedy dreams, and everyone was laughing.

In hindsight, the South Park episode was discouraging and inspiring at the same time. My friends were busting my balls, being supportive in their own rough way. If they had felt sorry for me and coddled me, it would have felt even worse. My friends knew I wasn't a simple stereotype like Timmy or Jimmy, but at the same time, it reminded me that even cutting-edge comedy could have old-fashioned views.

When you kick a ball over a fence, you can look through the slats and maybe see the ball, but you can't see the big dog lurking in the shade. I had hopped the fence to pursue the ball and was now painfully aware of the dog's presence. Before that night, I had a limited, naïve view of what it would be like to be successful, and I had blissfully forgotten the stigma of being disabled in popular culture.

I felt doubly resolved; I wasn't going to let that show derail my dreams. But I also couldn't forget that I had seen it. It was in my head. I learned a lot from it: 1) Disabled comedy was big enough to merit an episode of South Park, and 2) I would never be like Timmy or Jimmy, a disabled cartoon to be mocked.

A few nights later, Thor and I were sitting in his rowboat. "What are you going to do after you graduate?" he asked. "The big scary world is going to have fun with you." He giggled his creepy little laugh.

"It's funny you should ask," I told him. "I just figured out today that I'm going to Denver with my friend Liz. Her dad said he could get me a job at the—"

Thor straightened up. "Denver, huh? Listen, every four years I bump into a new Evergreen student in those woods." He pointed with his cigarette toward the beach. "The girl before you ended up leaving and moving to Denver, too."

"Hey, that's cool."

"I haven't heard from her since she left," he said. "You can find her for me."

"To be honest with you, Thor, I think that's a bit creepy."

He finished his beer and sucked his menthol down to the butt. And even though we were alone out in choppy open water, he leaned in and lowered his voice. "This is all hush-hush, by the way."

"Oh okay," I said. "I'm happy to go out and find this random girl, but what do I get out of it? Aside from the adventure?"

Thor looked into my eyes. "When I was a kid, my mom got a human skull from a garage sale. If I can find it, I'll give it to you."

"Deal."

For the next few nights, whenever I saw Thor, he'd divulge another detail about the woman he wanted me to find. "She's got a blue star tattoo on her neck," or "she's about your height, but shorter," or "she wears sandals a lot," always followed by "stand by for further information." I knew better than to simply ask for her name. Thor was too cryptic for that shit.

On the day I left Olympia, I went to Thor's house to say goodbye. I walked up his muddy driveway and noticed fresh animal prints. A gaze of raccoons was loitering by the door and scattered, skittering, at my approach. Thor came outside holding a manila envelope. He almost seemed surprised to see me.

"Today's the day, Thor," I said. "I'm going out into the big, scary world."

"I thought you were those damn raccoons." He looked down at the parcel in his hands, like he forgot he was holding it. "Oh, this is for you. This is your dossier. Everything you need to know about her is in this package, but don't open it until you cross the bridge into Oregon." The envelope was unevenly packed and awkwardly shaped. Thor gave me a hug and a wink. Then he forcefully tucked $30 into the front pocket of my jeans, mumbling, "For phone calls, or whatever." He stuffed a handful of pungent-smelling orange tree leaves and a Japanese two-yen bill into the pocket of my sweatshirt. "Always remember the unfortunate air hose incident," he said, nodding gravely down at his junk. I had heard this referred to quite a few times over the past four years. Anytime that his dick might come up in conversation, he'd say, "That was before the unfortunate air hose incident." I never asked him to elaborate.

"What am I supposed to do when I find this mystery girl?" I said.

He pointed at my chest and said, "You leave a hat on her porch."

"A hat?"

"She'll know what it means."

Liz and I were packed into her car with all our worldly possessions. I had met Liz when she served her tour of duty as my student scribe. She was immune to my animal magnetism, but because of this, we were able to become the closest of friends. I laughed with Liz more than anyone, and I was excited to follow her to Colorado. Not only did her dad have a lead on a job for me, she said he knew an agent who booked disabled comics. Looking back now, knowing what I know about the comedy scene, an agent for disabled comics works in a strangely niche market. I mean, really, how many of us could there be? But any small opportunity is giant when you're coming out of college trying to be a stand-up.

Five miles outside of Olympia, Liz turned to me. "You smell like oranges."

I took the orange leaves out of my pocket and tossed them onto the dashboard. I told Liz all about Thor and my mission. Her first question was, "So he's going to give you his mom's skull?"

"No. His mom has a skull that he's going to find for me."

"And you want that?"

"Well..."

"So, where is this dossier?"

For a moment, I thought I had lost it. We had so much stuff that the back seats were full and spilling into the front. I found the envelope wedged all the way in the back with a dried-up French fry and a hairy Skittle. I pulled the dossier out and showed it to Liz.

"Are you going to open it?"

We were nowhere close to the Oregon border, so to fill some time, I showed Liz the other random items Thor had given me. It turned out the bill wasn't Japanese yen at all, it was a Japanese peso. This was actually a very rare bit of currency from when Japan occupied the Philippines in WWII. Of course Thor would have some Japanese pesos.

Now Liz was as curious as I was about what might be in the dossier and urged me to open it early. I tore the top off with my teeth and was greeted with the distinct smell of skunk weed. I dumped the contents out: a five-pack of Scooby Doo pencils, followed by a baggie with a banana-sized bud inside. I opened the baggie and pulled the weed out. When I pinched it, I had a hard time pulling my fingers apart. For a guy who "didn't do drugs," Thor's weed was the nicest I'd ever seen in my life.

Liz wasn't paying attention. "I think somebody hit a skunk."

"It's this weed!" I told her, holding up the bag toward her face. "It smells like a skunk's rectum." I don't know why that should seem appealing, but my mouth watered when I said it.

The only other thing in the envelope was an ounce of psychedelic mushrooms. No photographs, no paperwork offering possible whereabouts or a physical description of this mystery woman. I tore the envelope apart to see if there were any further instructions written on the inside. Alas, there was nothing.

In all my years since, I never found Thor's mystery woman, and now I'm not so sure she ever existed. Just like the Easter Bunny.

OFF TO COLORADO

My first job after college was working as a counselor at an Easter Seals camp. Liz's dad Arnie lined it up for me. Easter Seals is an organization that caters to mentally and physically disabled people and gives them opportunities they might not otherwise receive. Liz drove me directly from Evergreen to the camp in Granby, Colorado.

I arrived two weeks late and missed orientation. I was wearing my favorite Cameroon soccer jersey: bright red, yellow, and green. When a guy like me is wearing a shirt that loud, people tend to notice, but there was nobody there to notice. We were in an empty, gray, gravel parking lot.

"I don't see anybody here," Liz said. "You sure this is the right place?"

"I'll be fine. I'll go find the main office and check in."

"You have everything you need?"

All I had was a beat-up, hiking backpack filled with my clothes, my drugs, my trusty soccer ball, and a machete from Senegal. "Yeah, I'm good."

She looked at all the stuff still left in the car. "Sure you don't want your George Foreman Grill or your bow and arrow?"

"Right," I said. "Hand me the bow and arrow."

We hugged it out, and Liz drove on down the mountain. I hoisted my backpack, grabbed my bow, and followed the wooden arrow-shaped signs to the main office. I left my gear on the wheelchair ramp outside; seeing how I was already late, I didn't want my new employer's first impression to be me prepped for the zombie apocalypse. I walked around, exploring the main building, but couldn't find anybody. The place was a ghost town.

Back outside, I ran across the gravel camp road and headed up the mountainside to get a better perspective. The mountain was steep and rocky, and the foliage was a lot different from Washington, much dryer. Everything was spiky. There were cacti and yucca and pine trees, none of the leafy greens of Olympia.

Forty-five minutes later, I burst out of the woods, covered in small cuts from all the new plants I had been acquainting myself with. Once back on the road, I encountered a large man, not entirely happy-looking. "You must be Josh," he said without a smile.

"Yes, I am."

"I'm Roman. The camp director." He studied me for a moment. "Where have you been?"

"Just getting the lay of the land." I should have had the machete and bow. It probably would have left a better impression.

"Did you bring anything?"

I led Roman back to where I left my cache of weapons. I could tell he wanted to say something, so I went on the offensive with a barrage of questions about the camp. I picked up my weapons with casual confidence, and Roman swallowed his objections. He told me to follow him and took me down to the basement of the main lodge where my cabin was. There were about fifteen bunk beds, and every other bunk had a hungover counselor sleeping in it.

Roman pointed. "Any open bunk is yours." He called out, "Remember everyone, the staff meeting is at noon. We have the craziest week of the summer ahead of us."

People fidgeted and groaned. It was just past eleven, sleeping in on their one day off a week. I found a place for my things while the counselors around me stirred and fumbled out of bed, muttering regrets about the previous night's drinking. After a round of lackluster introductions, I made sure my drugs were secure and left for the staff meeting. I was given two dossiers—real dossiers—on my duties for the week. These dossiers had everything anyone would ever need to know about the campers: height, weight, background, where they lived, names of guardians, photos, habits, and medications. I preferred Thor's version.

Ideally, there was one counselor for every camper, but that coming week we were short-handed. The thing I noticed right away was that both of my campers were described as runners. I understood the other behaviors listed in those packets: severe ADHD, hyperactivity, obsessive compulsion, schizophrenia. But runner was a new diagnosis to me. Honestly, it sounded fun.

When my first camper, Kyle, showed up, his guardian looked at me skeptically. I was younger and more disabled than he had hoped.

"Are you sure you've got this?"

"Oh, yeah. Sure. I've got it," I said, thinking back to all my experiences from Camp Sunrise. He left looking worried, but maybe, I imagined, relieved as well. Kyle was blond and scrawny, with a far-off look in his eyes. As we waited for my second camper, I followed Kyle to the light switch, which he compulsively flipped on and off, to the audible dismay of everyone else in the room.

Gabe showed up shortly after, a stout kid with a round, bald head. His guardians expressed the same doubt that Kyle's had.

"I can handle him," I said. "Really." As soon as the guardians were gone, I found out what a runner was.

As if they had planned it all along, Kyle ran out one exit, and

Gabe bolted out another. I stood there, slack jawed, wondering who to run down first.

My first week of work as a college graduate was as a marathon runner. I spent all my time trying to keep up with this dynamic duo. These boys could have powered the entire eastern seaboard with their hyperactivity. Even to this day, it was one of the craziest weeks of my life.

A fellow counselor saw the frazzled look on my face. "This is easier than last year. They tried to have severely disabled adults in wheelchairs the same weekend as these guys, and the hyperactives were pulling tubes out of people any chance they got. Now *that* was a nightmare."

"And you came back for more?"

Because I missed orientation, I didn't know anything about the layout of the camp. I didn't even know where to find a clock. If anyone told me to bring my campers to a certain place at a certain time, I was hopeless. Instead, I took the kids out into the woods and wandered with them for hours, hoping I could tire them out. Gabe was obsessed with haunted houses, and everywhere he looked, he saw werewolves and vampires. From the dossier, I learned that he had gone on a new medication the week before. I often considered eating a handful of Thor's mushrooms, just so I could be on the same level as my campers.

"There's a goblin!" Gabe would say. "Did you see that ghost?" he'd shout, pointing to a shadow in the corner. He couldn't sleep through the night and seemingly slept only four or five hours the entire week. One time, I woke up to Gabe trembling and pointing toward Kyle's bunk. "There's a dead woman in that bed."

"It's not a dead woman. That's Kyle." I was sleep-deprived

myself by then, being the one Gabe woke up when he couldn't sleep. "I agree. He looks dead. But he's not a woman. Please go to sleep, Gabe." I knew my words were useless; this would keep him up until dawn.

I learned I had to sleep on the floor at the foot of their beds to prevent Gabe from wandering off and looking for werewolves. There were fifteen campers in one room, and many of their counselors had to take the same precaution.

Kyle's thing was light switches. He incessantly flicked them on and off, on and off. If you let him, he'd do it for hours. And boy, did I let him. It must have really added to that haunted house effect. I realized fairly quickly I could use their passions against them. If they both went running, I grabbed Kyle first and put him in front of a light switch, then I went after Gabe. When we got back, Kyle was still there, manning the lights, and Gabe would be momentarily mystified.

By the fourth night, I was so strung-out from lack of sleep, I could hardly function. A counselor would sleep in front of the door to make sure none of the campers slipped out. I volunteered that night. In my delirium, I figured it would give me a chance to get more than two hours of uninterrupted sleep. I lay down and closed my eyes, and it seemed like I had just fallen asleep when I heard the sound of pouring water right next to my head. I opened my eyes to see a groggy boy standing over me, peeing. In one move, I rolled out from underneath an arc of urine, grabbed my shoes at the end of the stream, and ran into the bright hallway. A few seasoned counselors were already hysterically laughing at the spectacle of me and my dripping shoes. "Welcome to camp, newbie!"

"I quit," I said. "I fucking quit."

I didn't quit, I toughed it out. As the summer went on, I learned that every day a small thunderstorm rolled down the valley, usually about lunchtime. In the cafeteria during lunch, counselors marveled at the ease with which I spoon-fed my campers. I told them it was because our palsies canceled each other out. My joke was: "I'll feed you, now you feed me!"

It was all good until the storm was upon us. For some reason, the electricity in the air set off the smoke alarms in a quick burst of *barrr*, which in turn triggered all the palsy-startle reflexes in the room. All around the cafeteria, you could see spoonfuls of food flying up in the air, like confetti.

In the little free time we had, I would kick the soccer ball around with the other staff. One day, Erin, a fellow counselor with cerebral palsy, was watching the game and said, "You know there's a team for you, right?" She told me she was a Paralympic swimmer. I didn't even know what the Paralympics were until she explained it.

She told me that the Paralympics are the Olympics for people with physical disabilities, and it's the second largest sporting event on the planet. "I got to hang out with the soccer team at the world championships. There are some cute boys on the team, and they are fun to hang out with."

"Sounds like I'd fit right in." I replied, flashing my most charming smile.

"I actually have the coach's info. I'll give it to you." And she hobbled off to her cabin.

Two days later, she slipped me a piece of paper smaller than a gum wrapper, with the head coach's email. I folded it as carefully as I could and put it into my mostly empty wallet. I had no idea that such a humble scrap of paper was going to change my life forever.

◯◯◯

After I barely survived Easter Seals, Liz's dad Arnie and his new wife Amy took me in. I had given myself a rule when I went off to college: I would never go back to live with my parents. So instead, I went off to live with someone else's. They let me stay in the basement guest room of their house, which was nestled in the foothills of the Rocky Mountains, right outside of Denver.

I was eager to get started on my dream of becoming a stand-up comedian and wanted to talk to this agent who specialized in disabled comics. Arnie handed me a scrap of envelope that the agent had given him with his name and phone number. I waited until Arnie and Amy went to work and the house was quiet to give him a call. I didn't have a cell phone, and back then I was nervous to talk to anyone on the phone, worried they wouldn't be able to understand me. Honestly, I was afraid to even order a pizza, let alone speak with an agent who could launch my career.

The guy didn't answer the phone, and I left an awkward message, I'm sure he thought was some local comic pranking him. He never returned my call.

Then 9/11 happened. It was surreal living in a near-stranger's basement—I hadn't even unpacked my belongings—while the entire world went through that dark time. Regular life shut down, and comedy was the farthest thing from anyone's mind.

I was grateful to be living with such a nice family, even if it wasn't my own. They let me invade their home, like the son they never wanted had come home from college. They were so patient with my freeloading ass and my ravenous, weed-fueled appetite. Once, Arnie brought home a lasagna from a work function, and I ate the entire pan while they were gone, like a real-life Garfield. Arnie couldn't believe it.

"That was going to feed my family for a week," he said with disgusted awe.

Amy came to their marriage with a ten-year-old daughter. I came to their marriage with a machete, a bow and arrow, and a hearty appetite. Despite my newly adopted family's kindness, I grew stir-crazy. I had nothing to do but smoke what was left of Thor's weed and wander the hills. My dreams of comedy stardom seemed farther away than ever.

A few weeks later, Liz and I moved to a house in downtown Denver, on bail bond row. Her dad had been leasing it as an art gallery that displayed work from disabled artists, and he let us take over the extraordinarily low rent. There were hundreds of hooks mounted on the walls where the previous art had hung, and I felt inspired to fill those hooks up with my own art. I had been dabbling in drawing using charcoal and oil pastels, and I began to create every day.

Even though my rent was cheap, I needed a job. Arnie hooked me up with an interview to work as a counselor at Support, Inc., a day program where adults who are mentally and physically disabled can be cared for. Since I never heard back from the comedy agent, I took the job. It was similar to the Easter Seals camp—every day was a new adventure. We would take them on trips to the zoo or the museum, and in turn, give their families a break. Due to my physical appearance and unique gait, onlookers could never tell who was in charge.

Off to Colorado | 167

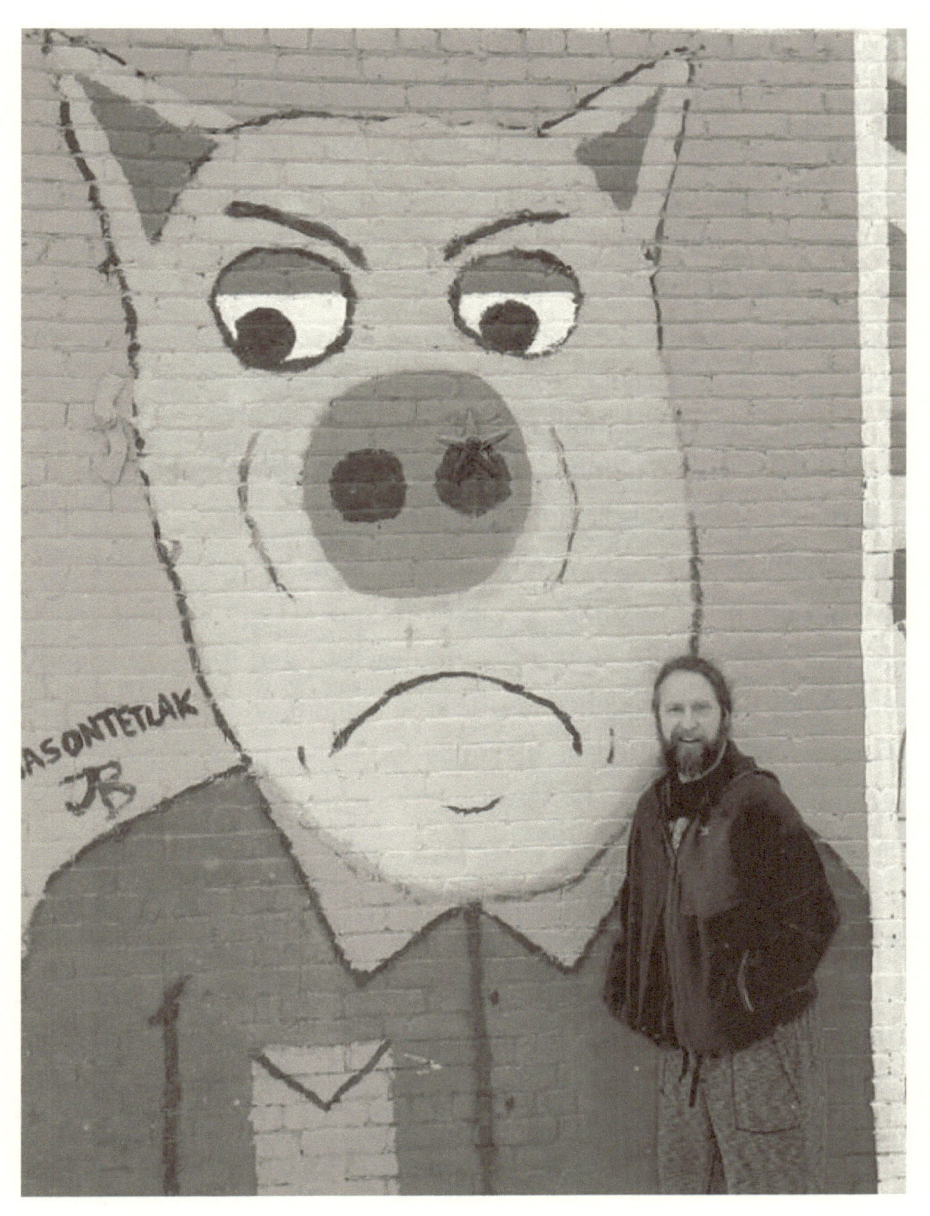

A mural I did later down the road of one of my notorious pigs.

Clients would start showing up at about 7:45 a.m., and I would generally get there at about 7:43 a.m., after a harrowing three-mile palsy bike ride through the city. The first task when the clients arrived was to check their diapers. I made sure to always look busy, and the entire time I worked there, I never changed one diaper. Eventually, a co-worker called me out on my dirty diaper dodging, and I replied, "I don't even like to wipe my own ass!"

I made quick friends with my co-worker Mike, who was in his mid-fifties and skinny as a scarecrow on crack; he'd wear tight jeans, and the ass was concave from the void. Our love language was talking shit to each other all day.

He saw me picking up dirty coins in the parking lot and asked, "Why are you picking up pennies?"

"It's money," I said. "Aren't we here to make money?"

After that, he would show up with a pocketful of pennies each day and scatter them on the ground like birdseed. I would eagerly pick them up. He laughed at the idiot picking money up off the ground, and I laughed at the idiot throwing money away. Plus, picking up pennies was one more way to look busy when it was diaper time.

One afternoon, I was supervising a handful of clients outside in our fenced-in patio area. A group of neighborhood teen boys would regularly ride by on their bikes, and on this day they stopped, mistaking me for a participant in the program and thinking we were unsupervised. They mocked and mimicked our movements and voices. In classic form, they one-upped each other with their hack cruelty, something I had dealt with since that first day at the bus stop. I had a thick skin and a sharp tongue from enduring decades of ignorance, but I felt especially angry for the fellow disabled people under my care.

The boys' laughter abruptly stopped, as something snapped in me, and I suddenly opened the gate and charged out. The booboo monkey was loose. The boys had foolishly assumed that I was a mentally disabled adult, not an angry 22-year-old who played soccer regularly and had no qualms beating up a 14-year-old. They saw the fury in my face and fumbled with their bikes, riding away in a screaming panic. I changed lives that day; we never saw them again.

()()()

I had been working at Support, Inc. for about two months at $10 an hour. It was a worthy job. It was a needed job. But I was going batshit stir-crazy. In my core, there was a voice telling me there's more to life.

Then they hired Brenda, and that voice turned into a scream.

From the get-go, she was a cheese grater on my existence. She talked down to the clients and to me as well, because she couldn't wrap her brain around the fact I was only physically disabled.

I remember all the counselors were sitting around talking about their education level during client naptime. Brenda bragged to everyone how she had just finished her two-year degree at a community college, then turned to me and asked in the deliberately slow cadence I have always hated, "Did you go to school, Josh?"

"Yeah. I just finished a four-year degree."

"Oh, really?"

I could see her trying to fathom the fact I had gone to college. I looked at Mike like, *what the fuck?* She was obviously treating me differently than the other employees.

I went to talk to my supervisor Pam about Brenda's condescending demeanor. Pam said she too noticed it. She called

Brenda in, and we had a sit-down meeting. Pam explained to her how I felt.

"I'm sorry. I didn't know you were perceiving it like that," Brenda said in her best fake-positive voice.

I kind of weakly smiled, and we shook hands on it. Pam dismissed Brenda, then said to me, "She's so full of shit."

Out in the hall, Brenda was waiting for me. "I'm sorry, buddy. I didn't know I was hurting your feelings. Oh. Is it okay if I call you buddy, or does that offend you, too?" Her tone made my skin crawl.

A week later, we were getting paired up with other counselors to take clients on field trips. I got paired with Brenda. She rolled her eyes and said to herself, "Ohhh. This'll be fun." Everyone heard it.

We took the clients to a cafe where she was a standoffish asshole to me the entire trip. As we were unloading our clients back at home base, she kept hitting me with snarky comments. After she saw she had visibly shaken me, she said, "Why don't you run and tell on me again?"

"Why don't you suck my dick?" I clamped my left hand over my mouth, as if to catch the words before they could escape.

I went straight to Pam and told on myself. "Brenda was being rude to me, so I said something to her I probably shouldn't have."

"What did you say?"

"I, uh, I told her to suck my dick."

Pam, as professional as she was, just started laughing.

Another meeting was promptly called with Brenda, and Pam told us it was time to squash this beef once and for all.

I offered Brenda an awkward apology. "Sorry I told you to suck my dick." It was kind of fun to keep saying it.

Brenda could sense Pam was not on her side, and she accepted the truce.

Shortly after that, word got to Brenda that I always had good weed, and she became very friendly to me. All my life I have noticed a pattern of people who don't take the time or effort to understand me, or disabilities in general, until it somehow benefits them, and then they suddenly treat me as an equal, if not better. If you genuinely change your opinion of me, I can genuinely change my opinion of you, but I do have a keen radar for bullshit. I extended an olive branch in the form of a joint, but Brenda had shown me her true colors, so I kept her at a crooked arm's length.

Two months after Brenda and I smoked our peace pipe, most of the staff took some clients on a trip to Las Vegas, leaving Brenda and me to care for the few clients who couldn't make the trip. I wanted to go, but it was a reward for senior staff members.

We were bringing the clients in, and I had just left Mark—a tall, eerily quiet, young man—inside and gone back out to the bus. I heard a woman shrieking and hurried back inside to find Brenda in a panic.

"Mark's killing Sonya!"

I handed off my client and ran into the main room to find Mark trying to kill Sonya. She was flailing on her back as he stood over her, raining down heavy punches. Mark was built like a pro tight end, but without thinking, I charged in, shoving him away from Sonya, and then stepping behind him to wrap him up tightly and lead him out of the room.

Something about the change in the daily routine had triggered Mark, but luckily, no serious damage had been done. After that, Mark was "my guy," and I was tasked with caring for him directly. Mark was very high-functioning, no diapers to change or special feedings, so the care was relegated to keeping him from trying to kill anyone else.

I would often take Mark out to explore Denver via city bus, as a way to both entertain him and explore my new home. We had free bus passes for the clients, but I would snag them for myself, too.

Pam cornered me one day. "Josh, you know those passes are for clients?"

"Well, I could be a client here."

I continued to take them.

One afternoon, as Mark and I were aimlessly wandering the streets of downtown Denver, we came across something that made me stop in my tracks: Comedy Works. I didn't know it at the time, but I was standing in front of one of the top three comedy clubs in America, if not the world. I wanted to go inside and check it out so badly, but we had to catch the bus back to Support, Inc.

()()()

Pursuing my comedy career was like courting a woman and the thrill of the chase. But now that I can look back, a comedy career is a long-term relationship. In a relationship, you love that person, but there are some trying times; it's not about changing the other person, but looking in yourself and adapting to new circumstances.

There was a time in my life when I didn't know if that relationship was going to work, or if any relationship would. There was a time when I felt like I had so much potential energy, but I was stuck in a rut of "what if?" You follow the trail down and wherever the road goes, that's where the rut goes. I watched disgruntled people around me stuck in this pattern, working a job they hated. I didn't want to be that, so I looked for ways to get out of it.

A lot of the time my thoughts turned to the darker side—how

to make money quickly without much work. *What if I am a good drug dealer?* Or maybe I could scam the elderly with my trademark impish charm. Panhandler, pickpocket, palsy hitman; I ran through the list of petty and not-so-petty crimes.

I thought back to my Vietnamese friends in Minnesota. In addition to the revenge trick with the giant mirror, they taught me a clever way to steal candy from the 7-Eleven: You buy a 64-ounce Big Gulp cup, cram it full of goodies, then top it off with the slushy of your choice. You pay 89 cents for the slushy, and walk out with $7 worth of candy. Although that was a clever trick, it didn't help me much as an adult. You can't pay the phone bill with a Now & Later.

In college, I dabbled in crimes ranging from pranks to felonies. I used to steal the one-liter bottles of Dr. Pepper at the campus deli. I would simply walk in, grab one, and then walk out like I owned it. I would steal ridiculous things from thrift stores just because I could. One time I went into a store not wearing a ten-gallon cowboy hat but left wearing a ten-gallon cowboy hat.

And then there were the mushrooms. Oh, so many mushrooms in college. Two of my friends, Hillary and Sarah, knew how to identify them. These mushrooms were called Blue Ringers, and they grew in freshly clear-cut forests. I ate a lot of those little beauties. I liked having my third eye forced open.

The ladies used to dry the mushrooms in old, empty pizza boxes. In mid-fall, there were pizza boxes from floor to ceiling, with an ounce of mushrooms in each one. I remember being more impressed with how they ate all that pizza than how they got the mushrooms.

Hillary and Sarah lived off campus, and I still lived on campus, so I was the logical connection to the dorms. We moved a lot of mushrooms one fall. We had the best deal on campus, a dollar a cap. They were so potent that when I sold them I had a disclaimer: "Never eat more than six if you want to stay on this planet."

The drug-dealing lifestyle progressed rapidly. I soon had a giant wad of cash tucked into a Star Wars pillowcase, and a shoebox full of mushrooms people were knocking at my door at all hours to buy. It scared me when I started getting people knocking at my door who didn't go to my school, saying things like, "I hear you're the mushroom guy." I'm a hard dude to miss as it is, but when you added the most intense mushrooms to the equation, it took my visibility to a new level.

A theater classmate of mine flanked me one day when I was walking through the quad. "Hey man, where did you get those mushrooms?"

This guy was usually intense, but now he was twitchier than normal, and his eyes were glazed with space dust from his return from Pluto. A few days earlier, he had come to me with $32, and as I painstakingly counted out thirty-two mushrooms, he received my usual disclaimer.

"I ate the whole bag," he blurted with a happy, far-away hollowness. "I tripped for two and a half days. There was a twenty-hour period where I was just going up." He kept talking, going into details only someone tripping balls could understand. After I had heard enough and tried to break away to class, he grabbed my elbow, and with deeply dilated pupils, asked, "Can I get more?"

Later that year, for his final performance piece, he did a whole monologue about Mrs. Butterworth. At the end, he stripped down naked out of his footie pajamas and poured Mrs. Butterworth over his hairy body in front of the whole theater class. As I watched, I felt responsible. This was clearly a ritual you could only learn on Pluto.

Just when the mushroom dealing started to get out of hand—and my roommate was sick of people knocking at the door around the clock—the season ended. If the supply had continued, I probably would have tried to juggle it, going down that road of easy money. With the money I did earn, I bought a mountain bike from a pawn shop. I loved that bike. It was my first big-kid bike. I loved it so much I had it shipped to Denver when I moved.

I knew I could make money selling drugs, but I wasn't ready to give up my comedy dream. I had that persistent voice in my head telling me there was more to life than this low moment.

Or it was just a flashback from those potent little mushrooms.

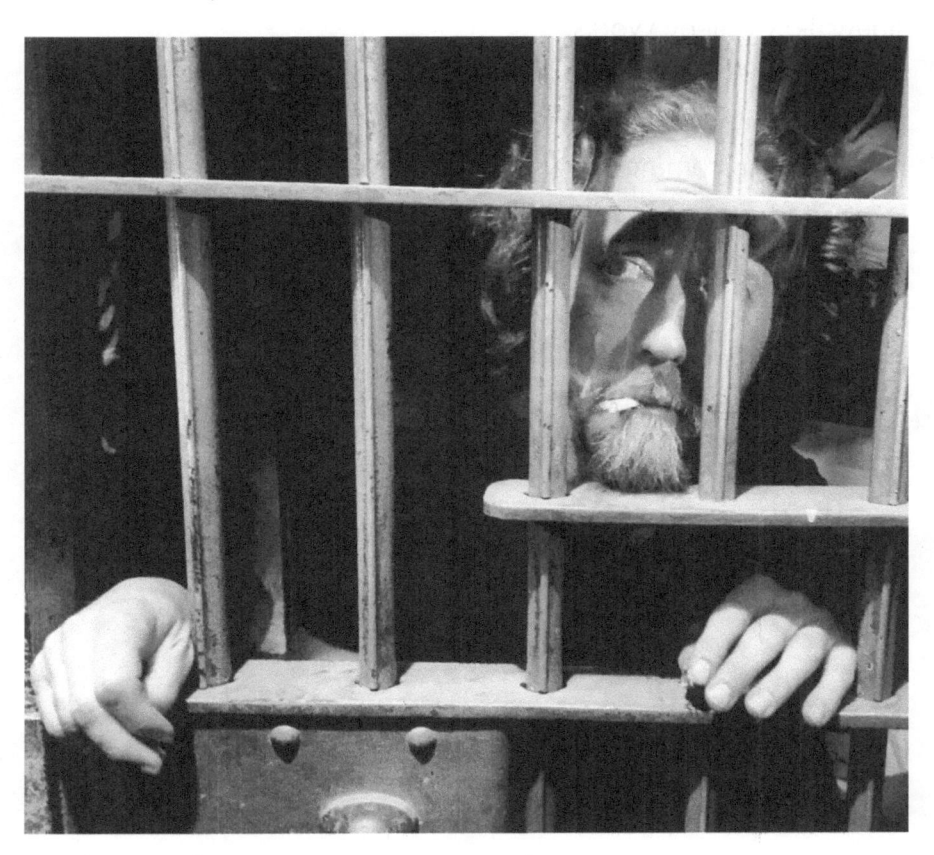

Me doing my best Paco impression years later.

Since my chance encounter with Comedy Works, the club called to me like a siren's song. I wanted to find the club again. No, I needed to find it again. I set out on a bright, warm day and headed north toward downtown. It's almost always sunny in Denver, and the sun makes the brick houses glow.

I knew the club was somewhere in Lower Downtown but didn't know the address or cross streets. This was still before the days of smartphones and Siri, so I was going on blind faith. It took a lot longer than I thought, and I grew frustrated. I was about to give up and head home when I turned a corner onto 15th Street and, *bam*, here it was, the black awning stretching over the sidewalk: Comedy Works.

All the doors were locked. I know, because I tried them all, I was desperate to do comedy again. I stood in awe, looking at the posters for upcoming shows. I didn't recognize all the names and faces, and that gave me hope. A couple walked up, arm-in-arm and really smiley, like they were in young love. I turned to them. "My face is going to be in one of these windows one day."

The corners of their lips went straight. They didn't frown or look skeptical. In unison, they said, "We believe you."

COMEDY ACT I

One beautiful Monday autumn evening, I was on what I thought was a date with a co-worker from Support, Inc. We were wandering around on the 16th Street Mall through the guts of Denver. My attention drifted from our conversation when I heard the telltale cadence of live stand-up comedy. I was drawn to a pair of speakers set up outside a bar called the Supreme Court. The voice pulled me to the open window where I saw a man standing under dingy lights performing to a less-than-empty room. I'm sure to my date it was one of the saddest scenes she'd ever witnessed, but it was exactly what I had been looking for.

After a moment, I turned to her and said, "I'm funnier than that guy."

She responded with the same indifferent shrug she had been giving all night.

I eagerly scampered to the entrance of the bar and asked the man checking IDs who was in charge of the comedy show. He rolled his eyes and flicked his thick thumb over his shoulder.

I don't know what I was expecting a comedy booker to look like, but it wasn't a man built like a fire hydrant, with hearing aids. Turns out this was John Raschke, the same agent I had been so nervous about calling from Arnie's house a few months ago.

"Can you put me on?" I asked, overflowing with confidence, my palsy making me dance in place. "I know I'm funnier than this guy."

"The show is already f-f-full," he said with a stutter and a wet sniff. "But I have a comedy contest every W-W-Wednesday at Ogden Street South. It's an open-mic contest. First prize is th-th-

thirty-five dollars."

If anything, this booker's disabilities filled me with more confidence.

"How do I get on?"

"You just sign up on a l-l-list."

Since I wasn't getting a spot, my date wanted to leave. I felt compelled to stay and check out the show but offered to walk her to her car, in the faint hopes of a goodnight kiss. After seeing my rabid excitement over the shittiest bar comedy one could find, she was fine going alone. We never went out again, although we remained friends at work. I grabbed a beer and watched the remainder of the painful performance. There were more comics than audience members that night, and Raschke introduced me to most of them. We were all clearly from very different worlds, but the one thing we all had in common was drinking.

The comedian I had heard from the street was Ron Ferguson, who eventually took me under his drunken comedy wing. I knew I had a passion to share jokes, but what I didn't know, and what my education at Evergreen hadn't taught me, was how to get gigs in the real world. I felt like I had so much potential, but if no one heard me, what was the point?

A few beers turned into all the beers, and I was fairly shitfaced as I shook Raschke's greasy meat steak of a hand again on my way out. I told him for probably the fiftieth time, "I know I'm funnier than these guys."

"All right," he said. "I'll see you on W-W-Wednesday. Get there ea-ea-early."

As I wobbled home drunk, my excitement for the Denver open-mic scene faded into regret: Did I really choose that ugly comedy crew over my date? I passed a random businessman and blurted out, "Hey man, am I destined to be alone my whole life?"

His timing was impeccable. Without skipping a beat, he answered brightly, "Yeah, probably."

That made me laugh harder than any jokes I'd heard that night.

By the time Wednesday arrived, I had rounded up everyone (six people) I knew in Colorado and showed up at Ogden Street South unfashionably early. I made up for it with the '70s pimp outfit I had assembled: a wide-brimmed hat, red bell bottoms, and a ladies' purple suede coat, complete with fake fur on the cuffs and collar. Raschke pointed me to where the list was. Three slots were filled, and twelve were empty. I signed up in the middle; my shaky signature covered slots seven and eight and half of nine.

Comics trickled in with audience members at a ratio of 3 to 1. The list turned out to be bottomless; come one, come all. I found out later that all the seasoned comics showed up at about nine-thirty, because they knew a Raschke room never started on time.

I felt like I was dehydrating through my sweaty palms, and the layers of non-breathable polyester I was wearing weren't helping. The show got underway. I felt like I was going up the first hill on a roller coaster, hearing the ominous *clink-clink, clink-clink*, wondering what I had gotten myself into. Some comics did well, and some were dismal; I hoped I could avoid the dismal column. Each joke a comedian told was like another *clink-clink* on the way up to Holyshitsville. This was what I had been dreaming of ever since I left Evergreen, but now that I was strapped into the roller coaster, the ride was a lot more real. I was far from Evergreen and my little insulated community.

The show was a grind, and even though I was in slots seven

through half of nine, it was clear Raschke wasn't putting people up in order, and every act was blowing past its five-minute time limit. My friend Liz approached me like a hostage asking to be released. I begged her for a little more patience—also she was my ride home.

I went into the bathroom and stood over the dirty sink, splashing cold water on my face. I stared at myself in the mirror, wild-eyed. "You can do this," I said to my reflection. "You're funny. You're a bad motherfucker." I adjusted my pimp coat and tightened my plastic belt. I heard a toilet flush in a nearby stall and exited quickly.

When I got out of the bathroom, Raschke was onstage introducing me. The roller coaster had reached the apex of the hill. I stopped worrying about what was coming. There was nothing I could do about it, so I threw my arms up and gave in to the ride.

"I'm a baaad motherfucker!" There was a rockslide effect to my opening line. By saying I was a badass, I knocked something loose. I started to believe it, and believing it helped me build confidence.

"Sleep with me now," I told the audience. "I'm gonna be famous." The crowd was laughing, but I couldn't be sure if it was my jokes, my outfit, or just the overall spectacle of the palsy pimp.

I wrote a setlist, but my handwriting was so illegible I couldn't read it. Instead of feeling the laughs and getting into a rhythm, I was trying to figure out what I was going to say next. I wasn't getting anything from that piece of paper I didn't already have in my brain.

"Sorry," I said as I fidgeted with the list. "I don't know what the hell I'm doing up here." That got a laugh, but the laughter wasn't as full. By calling attention to the sheet in my hands, I was taking attention away from myself. I was trying to hide behind my setlist and the ridiculous disguise I was wearing, but the brutal reality of being a comic is that the most you can hide behind is the microphone in your hand. You can't rely on anything else.

What I would come to learn is that the audience doesn't know anything until you tell them. By letting them know I was distracted by my setlist, I was highlighting my insecurity instead of just moving forward.

I came in there knowing I was going to win. I was definitely overconfident, especially for someone who had never even performed in the Denver scene before. Now that the show was almost over, I had to acknowledge there were a couple guys who might beat me.

Before Raschke announced the winner of the contest, there was a headliner, a professional from Comedy Works. The guy crushed, and he seemed like the very model of success I was looking for. Little did I know, he was barely scraping by, like so many comics.

While I watched, pounding beers and stewing in suspense, several other comics and a few patrons told me they thought I was going to win. I was even more confident in my chances.

When Raschke took the stage to announce the winner, it was well past midnight, and my guests were visibly annoyed. I wasn't going to be content with third or second, and when third place was announced and it wasn't me, I felt a wave of relief.

"Second p-p-place," Raschke said, and his stutter made the ceremony even more suspenseful. "Josh Blue." The audience reaction seemed split between regular applause and jeers that I had been robbed.

182 | *Something To Stare At*

The guy who won first wasn't even one of the comics I would have put in the top ten.

Offstage, when Raschke handed me my winnings—a beer and twenty bucks—he tried to console me, "You did g-g-great for your first time. You probably shoulda w-w-won, but he b-b-brought more drinkers."

He invited me to another contest he booked, and I was excited for another chance to learn from my mistakes and get the win. Just like when you get off a roller coaster, I wanted to run right back to go again. Prior to meeting Raschke, I didn't even know comedy competitions were a thing, but they played perfectly into my competitive nature.

"I r-r-recorded your performance. I'll get you the tape n-n-next week." That became my first demo tape, and the beginning of a long friendship with Raschke, who eventually became my off-and-on assistant.

Looking back, I'm sure I was never the badass I insisted I was in that bathroom mirror. The guy in the pimp suit was a character to cover up for how insecure I really was. I was playing a role to overcompensate for even a perceived lack of confidence. Between the stage fright and being self-conscious about my palsy, I wanted to project a level of confidence that was undeniable. After a few more shows, I packed away the pimp suit forever, realizing I was funny regardless of what ridiculous outfit I wore. When I perform now, I am the same person onstage as I am off.

()()()

I was going to shows almost every single night, even if I wasn't booked on them, to watch the comics and drink with them until the wee hours. Somehow, I was also able to show up at

Support, Inc. every morning. I came to find that Denver had a deep comedy scene. I was doing well and making friends, and other comics would feed me bits of info. What I wanted more than anything was what every up-and-comer wanted: to get a set at Denver's crown jewel—Comedy Works.

The sign-up for the open mic at Comedy Works was done with an automated phone line. You had to call a few days ahead of time and leave your name; then you had to call back on the day of the show and listen to a painfully long recording listing the lucky comics who would be performing that night. The rumor was that there was a six-week waiting list. The second week, I heard my name, and my heart skipped two beats. I remembered the posters I had seen in the windows that first night I discovered the club. This was where legends performed.

When people ask me to describe my show, they ask how much is scripted. I compare it to looking at a brick wall where every joke is a brick, and the improv is the mortar.

In college, I was the only person doing stand-up on campus, so I had no frame of reference. I would take the stage and do an hour by myself, without an opener or even an introduction. I would do new material each week, because the majority of the audience had been there the week before, and I couldn't possibly say the same thing to them.

In Denver's open-mic scene, I had five minutes at the most, and it went by in a flash. I had to learn to condense my longer stories into bite-sized bits. The open-mic recording stated new comics got two-minute sets, which was even more daunting. At that stage in my career, I felt better with the mortar stuff, riffing and improvising, but with only two minutes, I couldn't rely on the whim of the audience. I started to form my comedy brain. Before, I had a funny brain that could see the humor in things, but now I was looking at joke structures and the art of delivery.

Finally, that glorious Tuesday night arrived. I don't remember a single word I said, but I remember the big laughs. I felt like the King of the World after my first New Talent night. I came up shining in a sea of twenty-five comics. If laughter is a currency, I was barely earning minimum wage in the Raschke rooms. This two-minute set in a real comedy club was like robbing an armored car.

As good as I felt about my set, I knew I could do better. There was so much room for growth. The amazing thing about stand-up is you can never learn it all. Whether I was performing or not, I would go to Comedy Works and watch, just to learn other aspects of the machine. Many comics came in, did their set, and bounced. I never understood that. There was so much to absorb simply by being there.

So I ran back to the front of the roller coaster line again. I called that number every week, and for a while I was getting lots of stage time, almost every week. Then it dried up without explanation. I didn't know what was going on, but I knew laughs, and I was getting more laughs in my two minutes than some of the professional comics were getting in their five-minute sets at the end of the show. I couldn't understand why I wasn't getting called back.

The New Talent night at Comedy Works was run by Champagne Tuckerman the Last (not his real name), a middle-of-the-road veteran comic. He held the key to people's move up in the club. The path from little Tuesday-night spots to the big, paid weekend spots opening for legends like Brian Regan, Jim Gaffigan, and Dave Chappelle went through him.

Champagne Tuckerman the Last was the sole authority for who was on New Talent night, and he was no longer putting me onstage as often. The servers told me he saw me as a threat, because I was already funnier than he was. Over the months, I had become more than a new comic at Comedy Works. I had become friends with the staff. They embraced me as one of their own. I was soon not only one of the first to arrive, but one of the last to leave, after shift drinks.

I was stumbling out of the club one night when a seasoned server asked me, "Josh, you know why you fit here so well?"

"Nope," I answered.

"You get it. You're funny, you're respectful, you stay out of our way, and you tip well."

"Aw-shucks."

I learned how important and influential the servers are at a comedy club because they see it all. If you're not one of those four things he mentioned, they won't give you the time of day. If you're not on the servers' radar, you're definitely not on the owner's radar.

Champagne Tuckerman the Last had the power to control how often I got onstage at the club. He could have cultivated young talent. Instead, he discouraged me, hoping I would give up and fade away, like we saw him do with other promising new comics.

Finally, I got another spot. It had been a month since I was onstage at Comedy Works. I was given two minutes somewhere in the middle of the lineup, and I was ecstatic to be back there on the biggest comedy stage in town.

I was leaning against a pillar in the showroom, the only place left to see the show. I learned to watch the comic in front of me;

calling back one of their jokes was a great way to get the audience instantly on my side.

Between waves of laughter, Champagne Tuckerman the Last scurried up and whispered to me, "You need to move. You're blocking the waitstaff."

For as long as I could remember, and ever since, comics stood at that pillar and watched the show. Anyone with any awareness of the staff could easily step aside and let them through. I wasn't blocking the waitstaff, and everyone knew it. I pointed out other comics doing the same thing. "What am I doing that's different than anyone else here?"

"You need to move."

With a defiant sigh, I left the pillar and pushed my way through the nervous comics clogging the hallway backstage. As I rounded the corner, I looked over my shoulder and saw Champagne Tuckerman the Last had posted up in my exact spot against the pillar. That gave me more fuel; I was going to take that energy onstage and crush it.

The frantic emcee pressed me for my introduction.

"The comedian who puts the 'cerebral' in cerebral palsy," I told him. That was my standard intro for way longer than it should have been, because I thought the audience needed a heads-up. It was just another safety blanket.

The two minutes flew by, and I left the stage with a partial standing ovation. I was greeted with high fives and handshakes from the other comics. I looked for my comedian buddy and mentor Scott Johnson, a bearded bear of a man who usually watched my set and critiqued it for me. I found him getting an earful from Jim, still standing next to the pillar. I blew by, seeking praise and advice from other quarters.

Scott found me by the back bar. "Hey buddy," he said, "Champagne Tuckerman the Last says you're never going to make it 'cause you have no social skills."

My blood boiled. Lack of social skills is often unfairly attributed to people who are physically disabled.

Seconds later, Champagne Tuckerman the Last came around the corner with a fresh load of shit for me. "I need to talk to you in private," he demanded, barely masking his anger. He led me into the empty area where crowds would wait for a show to start and backed me into the cold rock wall. "First of all, good set," he said, to get it out of the way. "Second of all, you need to show me more respect."

Get fucked. But knowing he had the keys to my stage time at the club, I focused on keeping my composure.

"When I tell you to do something," he said, "you do it. You're not going to succeed in this business if you don't respect me."

I was high from the adrenaline rush of my set, and the tension was too much. My body began twitching like a live wire. "So what you're telling me is, you want me to kiss your ass until *you* think I'm ready?"

Champagne Tuckerman the Last closed the already short distance between us until we were nose to nose like boxers at a weigh-in. "That's not what I'm saying." He jabbed my chest with his finger. "You need to show me more respect!"

"Do you not like me for some reason?" I asked.

He started ranting. I had trouble following everything, probably due to my lack of social skills. If I could have backed up, I would have. I felt two milliseconds away from palsy punching him. I visualized the uppercut that would make his teeth clack together, hopefully catching some tongue. Before I popped him, I looked around for witnesses. Through a glass partition, I saw Christie, the manager on duty, with a concerned look on her face.

I understood if I punched Champagne Tuckerman the Last, I'd be done at Comedy Works. Christie was watching us, trying to figure out which one was the fool. I relaxed and let Champagne Tuckerman the Last carry on with his temper tantrum.

When he finally stopped, I said, "Can I ask you another question?"

"No! You may not ask me another question!" He turned and pounded away.

I stood there, stunned.

"What the hell was that?" Christie asked, snapping me out of it.

Shaking more than usual, I explained the best I could. Then I went up the stairs to the street level to get some fresh air and vent to the smokers.

The next day there was a big stink at Comedy Works, and two days later Champagne Tuckerman the Last was fired. I was promoted to the Almost Famous list, which meant seven minutes on weekend shows.

Looking back, I see what a crossroads that was for my comedy career. Had I lost my temper and knocked some of Champagne Tuckerman the Last's teeth out, my life would be very different today. Many opportunities in my life have come from being affiliated with Comedy Works and their great team.

◯)◯)◯)

A few months later, I signed up for the annual Comedy Works New Talent Contest. This was the highest level of comedy competition in Colorado, wherein hundreds of comics would pay a $25 entry fee and get whittled down to one winner over the course of the summer.

Winning the contest wasn't just about the $500 prize. Winning the contest was about bragging rights as the best among the up-and-comers, not to mention the winner was all but guaranteed to make "the list." Being on the list was the final promotion; it meant you got paid to open on weekend shows. The list was akin to being a Made Man in the mafia. You're officially in the family.

Every week there would be a showcase of fifteen contestants and from each weekly group, three would advance. I kept advancing. I ended up in the finals with eleven strong comics. All the performers drew numbers out of a hat to see what the order would be. Drawing numbers was nerve-wracking. You wanted a higher number so the audience would be warmed up and the judges had other comics to compare you to, but you wanted to avoid the dreaded tab drop. It's a notoriously distracting part of the show when the servers drop the bills, and the audience is trying to do drunken math. I pulled number eleven, which was ideal.

The showroom was packed. The energy in the room was crackling hot. It hit me that this was the most pressure I had been under so far in my comedy career. Time does a weird thing when you're waiting to perform in a contest: It moves both painfully slowly and dreadfully swiftly all at once.

The tabs were dropped and paid. People were focused back on the show. As I looked in the bathroom mirror, I felt like I was standing on the edge of a cliff, ready to take off in flight or plummet to my death. I gave myself the usual pep talk. "You're a bad motherfucker, and this contest is yours to take." The thing I was most worried about was a new joke I had thought of the day before. I liked the joke, but it's always a gamble to bring out an untested joke in front of a contest audience.

At last my name was called, and I took the stage with unmatched energy. I was not just performing, I was thoroughly enjoying the moment. The five minutes went by like a flash. I took a big chance by closing with the new joke. It turned out to be the strongest joke I had written to that point.

"I ride the city bus. And there's always one crazy person on the bus. Let me tell you something, folks. It was a sad day when I realized it was me! You see folks, I went to school on the short bus. And on the short bus, if you want to smear poop on the wall —it's okay! And if you want, pull it out." I swung the mic down between my legs, let it swing back like a pendulum, and then caught it when it came back up to riotous applause. "It's okay!"

The crowd roared for more. The hallway was filled with other comics who now knew they were hunting for second and third place. They shook my hand with "Great set!" Everybody, that is, except my buddy Matt Conty, who was the last performer of the night. He was paler than usual. As Matt was introduced, he walked past me and said, "Hey, thanks a lot, dude." Which, as everyone knows, really means, *you little motherfucker*.

When the crowd finally settled, Matt delivered what I thought to be the best line of the night. He spoke in his trademark deadpan style, "Every morning I wake up, and I thank God I don't have a disease like cerebral palsy, but tomorrow…I don't think is gonna be one of those days."

After tallying the votes, they announced the three winners, and I will save you the suspense: I won. The five hundred bucks and bragging rights were officially mine. I partied the night away with my co-comics. Even though I had all that cash, I didn't have to buy one drink the entire night.

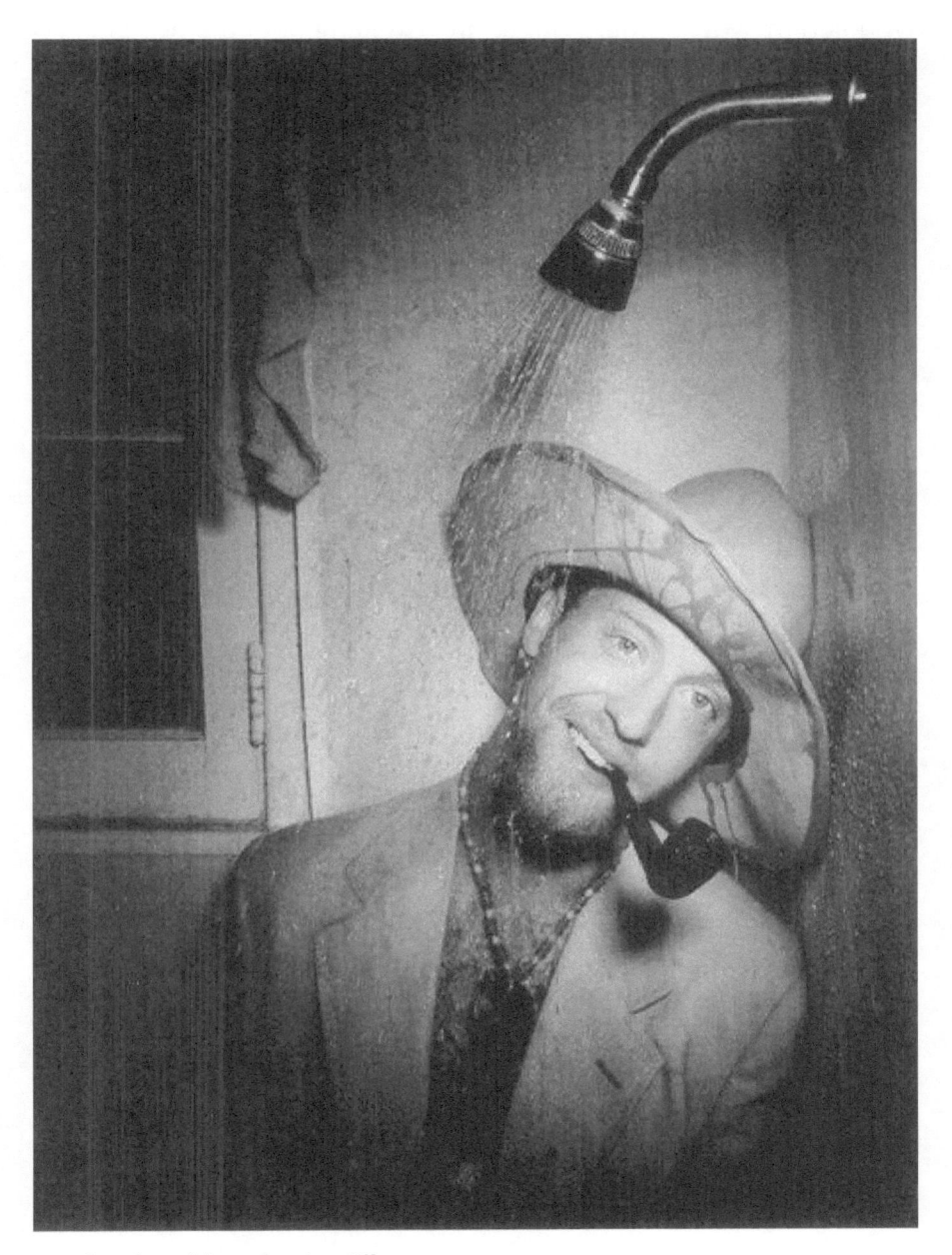

My first headshot, by Art Silk.

When the bar kicked us out, I was drunk as could be and wobbled my way home. With all the excitement of the evening, I'd forgotten to eat, so I was extra drunk and needed a greasy food sponge to absorb some of the celebration. I stopped by my local Taco Bell, which was the only thing still open, but only the drive-thru was available. There was nobody in line, so I walked up to the window and knocked on the glass, which they refused to open.

"Can I get some tacos?" I yelled at the closed window.

She responded like I was not the first drunk homeless guy she'd told this to. "You need a car."

"Please." I begged. "I just need two hard shell and two soft shell. I have money!" I said, holding up and fanning out my twenties. They were not impressed. I walked the rest of the way home, grumbling about what good is being a winner if I can't get any stupid tacos.

I became a permanent fixture at Comedy Works. I watched many comics at different stages of their careers, from beginners to A+ stars and performers sliding back toward a day job. I learned how a comedy club runs.

Rule number one: Stay out of the servers' way. They have more power than you know. A server plays a huge role in the forward movement of a young comic. It's common wisdom in comedy that if the servers are paying attention to your act, you're doing a great job. These people see comedy nightly, sometimes for decades, so if you can hold their interest long enough to make them laugh, you're saying something they haven't heard before. I distinctly remember the first time I noticed the staff coming out of the kitchen to watch me.

Rule number two: Don't go over your time. If you've got two

minutes, do one fifty-eight. Save those extra two seconds for the standing ovation. Over the course of my career, I've watched comics repeatedly go over their time—new talent and headliners alike—and they piss everybody off: the servers, the other comics, the management, even the club owners. The perfect time for a comedy show is ninety minutes. It's scientific. Much over that—and I don't care who you are or how funny you are—your audience needs to stretch their legs, they need to relieve the babysitter they're overpaying, and most urgently, they need to use the goddamn bathroom. There's only so much comedy club food your colon can handle.

Rule number three: The comedy club is a community. We don't have a union looking out for us, so we have to have our own code of ethics. Be cool to each other, don't undercut other comics on gigs or rates. And don't even try to sleep with the staff.

Rule number four: Be funny. It may seem strange that being funny is this far down on the list, but I've seen people become successful comedians by following those top three rules, and I've seen brilliant comics go nowhere because they don't know how to respect the community.

More than anything, I feel like the most important ingredient to becoming a comedian is having an active imagination. Part of that skill set is making your imagination relatable, so it's accessible to the masses.

I got to a point in my life where I didn't need to steal anymore. The rent at the Delaware House was $375 a month for the whole house, and there were three of us living there. I was getting a government check, and I was getting good money doing a smattering of college gigs and a bunch of local shows.

I was on my way to one of those shows at Comedy Works. It was a twelve-minute bike ride from my house to the club. I never wore a helmet for the lame excuse I couldn't buckle the chin strap. I probably should have worn a helmet walking; riding a bike was terrifying to me, and to onlookers, I'm sure.

Instead of pedaling through town, I rode along the Cherry Creek, a pleasant oasis in the thick of the city. I would push myself to pedal as fast as I could, like training for soccer.

Other people would get to Comedy Works ten or fifteen minutes before a show. I would usually get there thirty or forty minutes before. I don't know if the waitresses thought I was overly enthusiastic or a dumbass, but it gave me time to soak it all in, from the preparation of the staff at the club to the anticipation of the gathering crowd. It also gave me an opportunity to eat some food. My ritual was to meet other comics at a little deli near the club. I would lock my bike to the awning of the Comedy Works sign and study the faces on the posters of upcoming shows. I had started to develop a name, but my face still wasn't on the wall.

The deli was the closest food I could afford that tasted like my mom's home cooking. On this particular night, I felt like I could afford more than water with my meal. I decided to get a Gatorade to hydrate after my intense twelve-minute bike ride. The little orange rectangle price tag on the lid said $3.78, and to me, that was highway robbery. I paid for my Italian sausage and mashed potatoes; I didn't mention the over-priced Gatorade I had set on the table already. I wolfed down the meal that wasn't prepared on a single burner and triumphantly sipped my free Gatorade.

I strolled back to Comedy Works full and hydrated. When I rounded the corner of 15th and Larimer to the front entrance of Comedy Works, my drug-money bike was gone. It didn't dawn on me right away because they had even stolen the lock. The first thing that flew into my head was, *Karma is real*. I didn't need to steal that Gatorade; I did it because I could.

Ever since then, if anything of mine gets stolen, my opinion is that they needed it more than I did.

I was at another Raschke room, collecting another $30 prize for winning another contest. Between gulps of Budweiser, Ron Ferguson asked me to do some guest spots, opening for him on the road. At that time in my life, going on the road was an experience I had been coveting, a side of the business I knew nothing about: from booking to lodging to writing it all off on my taxes.

I greedily accepted Ron's offer. I thought about my day job at Support, Inc., and how I was going to strategically use the three sick days I had. "By the way, next Wednesday through Friday, I'm going to be sick."

"That's not how sick days work, Josh."

The tour was in Wyoming and, winding through the mountain passes in Ron's little red pickup, I found a Chris Fonseca CD buried in the fast food trash around my feet. "Hey, I studied this guy in college."

"I open for him on the road sometimes," Ron said.

Fonseca needed to work with a comedian willing to drive him, and I realized I needed to have the same service. It was cool of Ron to bring me, since I don't contribute much as a co-pilot. I can't drive, I can't read a map, and I can't put a CD in the stereo without scratching it. Ron invited me just because he liked my comedy, and we had a great time together. Either that or he was trying to fuck me.

Now Chris Fonseca wasn't just some guy I had studied in

college. This was a guy who had been in Ron's truck, in the same seat that I was sitting in. I had taken this little tour without many expectations and suddenly realized I was following in the buttprints of someone I had looked up to.

I started to put the Fonseca CD into Ron's heating vent, and he snatched it away, amused, and put it in the right slot. Track one started to play, and I was all ears. As the Wyoming landscape slipped by, we took breaks between laughs to remark on his well-written material. Fonseca trains you to listen, because you know you'll be rewarded with a laugh. You're willing to listen, to labor to listen, because you know what's coming is going to be worth the effort.

That night, our gig was at a high-end restaurant whose specialty was exotic meats, like ostrich, reindeer, kangaroo, emu, anteater, and many other animals you can find at the zoo. I sampled them all, and I have to say, gentle reader, my favorite was the dolphin. It was a strange place for a comedy show, and it was damn near empty. I would soon discover why—the headliner was a ventriloquist, in my opinion, the lowest form of comedy, followed by magicians and prop acts.

Going on that little Wyoming run made me realize the show at the Supreme Court, where I had met Ron, wasn't that bad. And people weren't chewing on raw hunks of seal meat. The more I did comedy, the better frame of reference I had for good shows and bad shows.

The next morning we were speeding across Wyoming when a giant tumbleweed the size of a Volkswagen Beetle rolled out in front of us. Our truck went right through it, and it shattered like a wicker basket. We laughed for the next twenty miles. Ron wouldn't let me play the Fonseca CD again.

A year and a half later, on my way to the airport to do a well-paying gig, I saw the Wyoming ventriloquist driving a blue shuttle bus to the airport. His unhappy face made me realize how delicate and cruel a career in entertainment can be.

Support, Inc. was moving an hour-and-a-half bus ride away. I told them, "When you guys move, I'm done." By this time, most of my co-workers, including Brenda, had seen me do stand-up. They knew I was going to be just fine. I was the one most nervous about it.

I had saved a bunch of money. I was and am a man of simple tastes. The only bills I had were my ridiculously low rent, groceries, beer and weed, and the occasional pair of tennis shoes to replace the ones my right toe aggressively wore through walking back and forth to the comedy club.

Things don't line up like this without a reason.

During that painful tour of Wyoming, Ron told me that Chris Fonseca lived in Colorado Springs, about an hour south of Denver, and often performed around town. I was excited at the chance to meet him and possibly even open for him.

One night at Comedy Works, there was commotion with the door staff, as they scrambled to figure out who was going to carry Fonseca down the stairs. Much to my chagrin, the comedy club was not accessible—yet. However, this gave me an opportunity to meet him. I held the back door open for Fonseca with vibrating palsy excitement and said to him, "They really need to make this accessible."

When you meet one of your idols, you try to keep yourself in check, and you try to let them talk and not interrupt. It's a great opportunity to listen and learn. And remember, they're never as excited to meet you. Once he was down the stairs and situated, I approached him and extended my crooked hand. "It's an honor to meet you, sir." I said. "I studied you in college." I hoped my excitement wasn't coming across as ass-kissing.

"I was hoping to see you here tonight. I've heard good things about you. It's nice to see a fellow palsy person," said Fonseca.

Excited that he knew who I was, I blurted out, "We should do a show together sometime!"

Trying to be casual, I stuck as close as possible to him all night, hungry for any tidbit of info. As the night progressed, and Fonseca got wasted, he was less interested in dispensing advice and grew belligerent to anyone around him. This was not the person I wanted him to be, and I distanced myself.

Even so, I stayed and watched his show. He was hilarious. I laughed, and I clapped, and I hung on his every word, like the rest of the audience. I was in awe of how comfortable he was in that broken body. Despite our rocky start, Fonseca and I became not just friends but brothers-in-palsy, and now I can look up to him in that way I always wanted to.

In this business, the best accelerant for a career that is catching fire is a comedy buddy. Someone with more experience than you, and who has the same comedy standards. A friend who pushes you to do better. No matter how hard I crushed, I would come offstage, and Scott Johnson would be there to tell me, "Nice try, buddy. Maybe you'll get 'em next time." Of course Scott knew when I did well, but roasting is the love language of comics.

Scott is a big, gay bear of a man. He looks like a lumberjack out of the woods of Washington, all flannel and work boots. We enjoyed nothing more than getting high and making each other laugh. We fed each other with our dark humor, always pushing the other to say the next horribly funny thing. Scott had left his own blossoming career in L.A. to come root himself in the hot Denver comedy scene. He went from being a touring, headlining comic, to being the Comedy Works house emcee, and he was extraordinarily good. He is, to this day, the best emcee I've seen.

Scott was a verbal chainsaw. When he took the stage, he demanded your attention and respect. He was unafraid and unapologetic. He talked directly to the audience, calling out the meatheads and soccer moms from Highlands Ranch, the Denver suburb "where married people go to die." He taught me that when you host as an emcee, it's actually *your* show, like being the host of *The Tonight Show*. The audience sees you throughout the evening, and it should feel like you're introducing your friends.

Scott and I would take epic walks. The two of us were a spectacle, lumbering through the streets of Denver; one little, wobbly guy and a giant, wearing a little girl's pink backpack which contained a notebook, weed, and weed paraphernalia. We would drink coffee, laugh, and wander for miles, writing jokes I would more often than not see him put into the show the same night. He showed me you could take the day's experience onstage and puke it out for everyone to enjoy.

I had the opportunity to open for Scott on the road a few times. Our rapport onstage was playfully combative. Comedy Works caught wind of this train wreck and offered us our own eight-week series every Monday. We called it BoBo and Blue, and it was a golden disaster. There was a lot of drinking involved. We danced and drank onstage, then told jokes and drank some more.

The Denver comedy scene was exploding with new talent, on par with the worldwide surge in independent and alternative comedy. To be honest, I didn't like alt comedy; it seemed like wacky set-ups with no punchlines. My comedy is the classic model of set-up and punch, just jokes. But the freedom of alt comedy was exciting and opened the door to comedians producing their own shows. We would pluck newer comics we thought deserved stage time for the BoBo and Blue show. The catch? Scott and I never left the stage. We would sit behind this poor rookie and ruthlessly heckle them and, of course, drink.

It was a variety show, with stand-ups, sketches, and plants in the audience. Not every bit landed. On one of our first shows, we had a young Black comic sit front row in the audience. Then we had a White comic come onstage and say something vaguely racist. The Black comic jumped onstage and started whipping the White comic with his belt. On paper, it was hilarious, but in reality was terribly awkward for us and the crowd.

In another episode, there was a young comic desperate for stage time, but we weren't sure if he was ready. We told him if he could prove his dedication to the craft by letting me palsy punch him in the head onstage, he would get a set. He eagerly accepted, and, for his service, received a black eye and a woozy three minutes.

At the writers' meeting the next week, Scott said the show was fulfilling his perverse desire to puke on the audience's brain. Week after week we did just that and, as you might expect, puking on the audience's brain yields mixed results. But people kept coming to the show, a combination of word of mouth and the club's creative promotion.

Comedy Works had a limousine company sponsorship. They

provided us with a limo for a night to promote BoBo and Blue. Scott wore a WWII army helmet, and I wore a purple velvet coat, aviators, and a fedora—my old pimp costume from that first Raschke show that now seemed so long ago. We rode around downtown Denver, hopping from bar to bar.

We had thirteen other comics, and the Comedy Works staff crammed in with us; they all had disposable cameras. The limo driver dropped everyone but Scott and me off a block away from the next bar. We circled around the block while the group positioned itself in front of the bar as paparazzi. When Scott and I stepped out, the camera flashes popped off, and the women screamed, creating a buzz that was almost bigger than the one in my body.

The rule was one beer per stop, which turned into three. Scott and I wandered around the bar, shaking hands, and the fake paparazzi handed out flyers and said things like, "Oh, you don't know who these guys are?" This unconventional promotion worked, and soon the shows were selling out.

At every show we invited the audience to an afterparty at Nawlins, a friendly Irish pub a block away from the club. I was amazed at how many people came out. BoBo and Blue took over the entire bar. People showered us with praise, but I knew they weren't seeing me at my best.

Scott and I never had to buy a drink. One night, the server pointed out in her cute Irish accent, "Each of you has nine beers on back order." I opened Scott's breast pocket and poured my beer into it. He reacted by throwing the contents of his glass at my neck. Someone handed me a full one, and I dumped over his head. As he tried to avoid that, he slipped and fell on his back, which made it much easier to pour more beer on him. He laid there in a lake of beer as the same waitress came over and mopped up around his giant body. Through his laughter, he kept saying, "I'm sorry, I'm sorry." She smiled and tried to clean up the mess as I dumped another beer on him. She wasn't mad; she knew we were the reason all those people were there. She offered, "Looks like you're ready for those other beers."

Not until much later in life did I realize what a magical time this was; comedy was my full existence, and I didn't have any other responsibilities. There was no business side to worry about; I was doing shows for money, beer, or ideally, both. I have never felt like more of a rock star, even to this day. While I have since had many more national and even global accomplishments, there was something about this success at a local, intimate level that blew me away. I would catch people staring at me on the street, and for the first time it was for something positive—they were recognizing *me*.

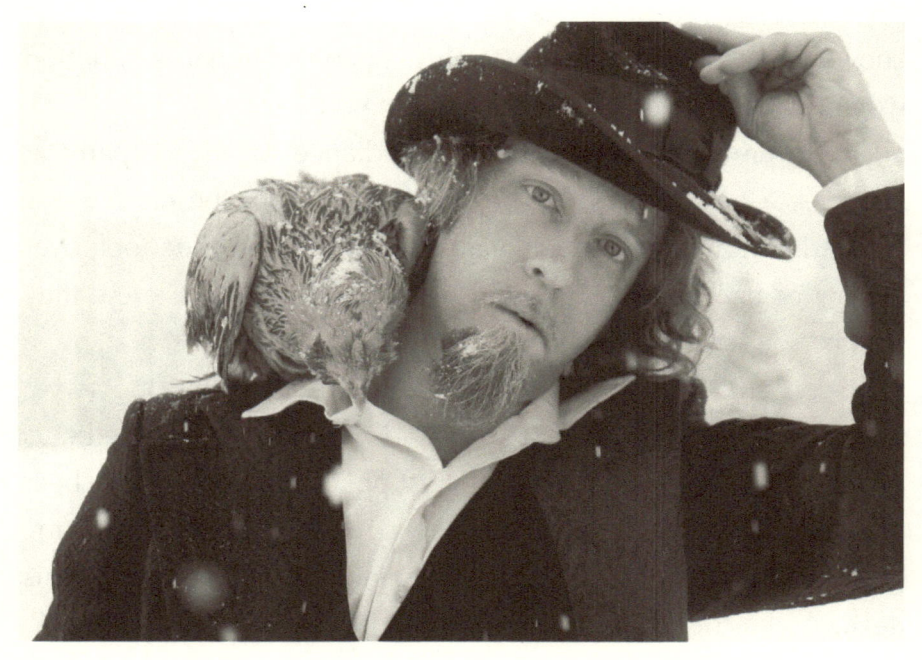

Another headshot of me with my cock out, by Chelsea Kuhn.

SOCCER

After this bit of success in the Denver comedy scene, my confidence was boosted enough to fish out that little, faded, soft scrap of paper from Easter Seals camp with the Paralympic soccer coach's email on it.

Hello my name is Josh Blue, I'm twenty-two years old, I have cerebral palsy, and I'm a damn good soccer player.

Without hesitation, I sent it off.

Much to my surprise, the next time I checked my email, there was a reply from the coach. Nervously, I read, "Hello Josh Blue, it's nice to meet you. We're always looking for damn good soccer players. We're having a tryout in Washington, D.C. in two weeks. We'd love for you to attend." Not only did they want to see me, they were going to fly me out on their dime. This was a far cry from getting cut from my middle school team.

Two weeks later, I was at my first training camp in D.C. The person on the other end of that email was U.S. Paralympic head coach Rick Moss, a short Englishman with a strong accent and a fun, warm energy. He showed up at our hotel room with two large bags of deflated soccer balls and a hand pump, and explained that as the new guy, my duty was to pump these up. He looked at my bright red, yellow, and green Cameroon jersey. "And by the way, you're wearing the wrong team's jersey."

Eager to fit in, I set to pumping.

"Welcome aboard." My roommate, John McCullagh, gave me a sly smile while lounging on his bed. He was an intimidatingly tall, bald man without any visible disabilities.

I had asked him about this earlier, and he told me he had an invisible disability, a traumatic brain injury he suffered while serving in the Coast Guard. He explained that in Paralympic soccer's own class system, you either had to have cerebral palsy, a brain injury, or a stroke to be on the team. John was a Class 8—the least amount of disability you can have and be on the team. He looked me up and down, "You'll probably be a five-six, which is the most amount of disability you can have and be on the team. A class seven is somewhere between you and me."

"Here, let me pump a few for you," he offered, as he noticed my pace was slowing.

There was a light knock on the door. I opened it to a large, shaggy man with a wonky arm.

John introduced us. "This is Josh McKinney. He's a classic seven. See how he's only affected on the right side?"

We connected our palsy hands in something that resembled the love child of a high five and a handshake. With a slight limp, Josh made his way into the room, gently kicking balls out of the way, and sat down next to McCullagh.

"Wow, you sure have that motion down," he said, watching John's rapid up and down pumping.

I laughed. This was another language I was fluent in—ball busting.

John finished with the ball, threw it hard at McKinney, then tossed me the pump. "Back at it, newbie."

"McKinney is our star player," John said. "He's a palsy guy like you, and he's the best seven in the world. In international play, you can only have two eights on the field, you have to have at least one five-six, and you can fill in the rest with sevens, if you have them."

"We only have two five-sixes on the roster now." McKinney said. That meant I only had two people to beat to make the team.

I finished pumping the last ball and juggled it to show off my skills, then lobbed it to McKinney, who headed it into my chest pretty hard. Thus began my long, long love affair with practicing soccer in hotel rooms, which is a great way to ensure you won't be getting your deposit back.

Later that day on the Paralympic pitch, which is smaller than a conventional soccer field, I was happy to see I wasn't the only one struggling to put my socks on. At least I could tie my shoes; there were some players who couldn't. I had replaced my Cameroon jersey with a brand new white and blue kit, complete with the official U.S. Team emblem.

Friendly faces invited me to kick the ball and warm up with them. Coach Moss blew the whistle, and we all gathered around. He officially introduced me to the team. "This is Josh Blue out of Denver. We're going to take a look at him. Seeing as how we already have a Josh on the team, we will call him Bluey." This was not a suggestion or a negotiation; when the coach handed out a nickname, it was done. I liked it. We should all be so lucky to have a great nickname like Bluey.

Before we jumped into it, we had a light warm up, where I quickly broke a sweat and ran out of breath despite the smaller field and the fact I was coming down from the Mile High City. *It's going to be a long camp if I'm already winded.* I tried to hide my exertion and sweaty blotches. It was blowing my mind that here I was, passing the ball with one of the best sevens in the world. And a day ago I didn't even know what a seven was.

On the field there was a ton of trash talking, as players made fun of each other's disabilities.

"Good pass, but let's see you do it with your bad foot."

"You run like a muppet."

Being surrounded by disabled peers was new to me, and the comfortable way they insulted each other made me realize these were my people, and in turn, made me want to make the team even more.

Halfway through the practice, we played a game where you had to steal the ball away from a teammate. Every new drill was a learning experience, because I grew up without the fundamentals. Most of these players had been on structured teams from a young age, but I had never been on a team since being cut in junior high.

It was my turn with the ball and I was heading toward a veteran player they called Woozy, short for Wobbly Woozy.

"Okay Bluey, let's see what you've got," he said, getting into a defensive stance.

I made a slight move right, and then a hard left, leaving Woozy on his back. I sloppily dribbled the ball to the end line. I turned and looked at Coach for reassurance. He was whispering to his assistant; I couldn't tell if they were impressed.

Toward the end of practice, I noticed two strangely familiar figures making their way toward the field. They were my sisters, Emily and Jessica, there to support me. I asked Coach if I could give them a hug.

"Make it quick, Bluey."

They reluctantly hugged me, as I was drenched in sweat. Their presence gave me an added burst of energy. I ran back on the pitch, and Jess called after me, "You're doing great, Bluey!" Despite my lack of conditioning, I finished the practice strong, fighting for every ball.

During the cooldown, we continued cracking jokes on each other. The goalie still had his oversized gloves on. I said, "Hey,

Mickey Mouse called, he wants his gloves back." Not my best joke, but everyone laughed.

From the side, the coach called, "I think you'll fit in just fine here, Bluey."

Getting Coach Moss's approval reassured me that I was in the running to make the team.

○)○)○

After four days of training camp, Coach Moss called me into his office, a.k.a. his hotel room. "That was a good first camp," he said. "You're doing things a five-six shouldn't be able to do. Your start-up speed is better than some of the eights, and you can stop and turn on a dime, which is not normal for your class. You definitely need to work on your fitness, though. Do you have a valid passport? We're taking twelve players to Holland in three weeks for the EuroCup, and I'd like you to be on the roster."

"My passport is valid, and I would be honored to be on the team. Not so sure about the fitness part," I said.

"I'll send you an email with drills you need to be working on," Coach replied.

I went back to my room, shaking with joy. Getting cut from that junior high team had been a miserable experience, but I never lost my love of the game. I had played whenever and however I could, dribbling the ball around the Evergreen campus, playing street ball with friends and pickup games in Senegal. Making the U.S. Paralympic team made that terrible moment in junior high suddenly so small and distant.

That night, the team went to dinner at one of the players' parents' mansion.

"Make yourself comfortable," they told us.

"You're lucky I'm not up in your bedroom, sleeping," I answered, without skipping a beat.

"Bluey says he's a comedian," Coach informed the hosts.

Relentless self-promoter that I am, I had a VHS tape of my comedy with me at all times, just in case. After dinner and a self-guided tour of the home and medicine cabinets, someone said, "Let's watch that tape, Bluey!" The dinner I had just devoured turned into a rock in my stomach. Cheers went up demanding the VHS. I didn't think it was such a good idea; there were little kids around, and parents. The footage was my first performance from Ogden Street South and riddled with profanity.

"Maybe we shouldn't play this in mixed company," I said as McKinney wrestled the tape from me. People gathered around the TV, and someone jammed the video into the player. I edged to the back of the room as Raschke's voice came up, "Coming to the s-stage, a n-n-newcomer, Josh Blue!" Groans and cheers came up from my new teammates as I staggered onto stage in my polyester outfit. That's when I left the room. I must have said *fuck* no less than forty times in a five-minute set.

I paced around their house while they watched. I could hear trickles of laughter coming through, hopefully in the right spots. Afterward my teammates piled on, letting me know that they thought I was funny, but now the door was off the hinges for shit-talking.

()()()

After three weeks back in Denver of non-stop beaming and bragging, I was back at a training camp with the eleven other cripples that were selected for Team USA to compete in the EuroCup. Why was the U.S. team allowed in the EuroCup, gentle reader? Because Paralympic soccer was so short on teams, they invited us to participate.

We went directly from the camp to a small town in Holland right at the border of Germany. My first stay in Europe and what an amazing way to go! A free trip with a national team. On the flight there, I daydreamed about the coach who cut me in junior high and wondered if any of his players had traveled to Europe on a national team.

Once we arrived, we had a few days to acclimate to the new time zone and get a few last practices in before our first game against Ireland. The day of the game, I grew more nervous as Coach told me I would be starting and playing midfield. I spent the time leading up to the game goofing around with my teammates and pretending I wasn't terrified. It reminded me of waiting to go up at the Comedy Works contest, but now the stage was global.

Before I knew it, the whistle blew, and it was game on. Again, just like with comedy, once I was out there, all the nerves left my body, and all that was left was the raw excitement and energy of the game. Paralympic soccer differed from conventional soccer in several ways. As I mentioned before, the pitch was a bit smaller, but the games were also an hour instead of ninety minutes. Teams were seven a side, not eleven. Throw-ins could be rolled in, and there was no off-sides rule, which was great for my lazy, cherry-pickin' ass.

Early in the first half, the ball came bouncing across the mouth of the goal, and I smacked it with my right foot into the back of the net. My teammates and I went nuts. I ran to the corner flag and did a little palsy disco dance. At halftime it was still 1-0. Toward the end of the game, I was exhausted and running solely on adrenaline. I had not spent the last three weeks working on my fitness, as the coach had suggested, and now I wished I had.

In the second half, Ireland tied it up 1-1. Then I was dribbling down the right flank, about twenty-five yards from the goal, as the defender moved to shut me down. I saw McKinney breaking for the goal and kicked a cross toward him, hoping his head would find it. Instead, it went into the upper-right corner of the net, never to be touched by the goalie or anyone else. It took me a second to realize I had scored. Only when I saw everyone on the field staring at me with slack-jawed amazement, teammates and opponents alike, I jumped the highest I'd ever jumped. We won the game, and I was hailed as the new break-out phenom. I never told anyone that I was just trying to pass.

Coach caught me on the back and asked, "Did you hurt yourself celebrating? I swear I've never seen anyone jump their own height before."

For the rest of the tournament, all eyes were on me.

When we weren't playing, we were watching the other teams, and I thoroughly enjoyed hanging out with the European players. The Scottish and the Irish had a deep-seated hatred for the English —not sure why. I think it had something to do with that movie *Braveheart*. When the English team would take the field, the Scottish and the Irish would all stand and sing together, "Stand up if you hate the English, stand up!" My other favorite was when someone would kick the ball out of bounds, everyone in unison would sing, "Are you English in disguise?" and then bray like donkeys. It was great fun, and it became our advantage, because we made it to the finals against England. Even though we beat all the other teams, they were rooting for us over the English dogs.

The English team was shorter as a whole than the U.S. team, but they played fiercely. There was nobody on our defense who was under six feet tall. The English star player's name was Woody, a stumpy seven. He barked orders and kept the team tight, but somewhere in the first half, we were able to break through their defense and score.

At halftime, Coach said we were playing well, but it was going to be difficult to hold that lead. "Come on, lads, only thirty more minutes."

We came out in the second half playing cohesively as a team, but the English were still able to tie the game early in the second half. The last twenty minutes were exhausting. We battled back and forth, and each team had a few shots on goal. When the whistle blew at the end of regulation, it was tied 1-1. Back on the bench, my legs were jelly.

"Come on, Bluey, I want to see you jump your own height again. Whoever scores here wins it. Sudden death," Coach said.

Back on the field, I could tell the English were just as tired as we were, but we had the crowd's shared hatred of England on our side. The ball changed possession several times, then Woody had a break down the right side of the field, barreling toward me with the ball. He made a move left, but I was able to toe-poke it off him. I settled the ball and then booted it back to big John McCullough on defense. He one-timed the ball forward, high and up over everyone's heads, to Josh McKinney, who was all alone about twenty yards from the English goal. McKinney trapped the pass perfectly and moved in for the kill. The look on the goalie's face was that of a doomed man headed for the gallows. McKinney smacked the ball into the back of the net, and the goalie didn't have time to move his feet.

We all screamed and chased after McKinney; he ran around and made a large arc on the field, and ended up sliding on his belly in the center circle. We all pig-piled him. Somewhere in the celebration, I realized I do not like pig piles.

That night, there was an awards banquet where we received our trophies for winning the tournament. We were the first United States men's national team to win a tournament outside of the U.S. I could tell it stung the other teams to lose to the Americans guesting in the EuroCup.

After the banquet, all the teams went to a bar and got annihilated. Somewhere between beers number four and thirty, the Irish coach, who had formerly played as a five-six goalie, wobbled up to me. He was bald and had a positive intensity about him.

"Bluey, you're a compliment to your class," he said in a thick, drunken, cerebral palsy Irish accent. "You're very good. Everyone was focused on defending you, when they should have been worried about McKinney."

The rest of the party was a blur. At some point, I got my ass grabbed by a Dutch player everyone called Harry Potter because, well, he looked just like Harry Potter. Some of his teammates told me he was sweet on me. I spent the rest of the night moving around the bar trying to avoid a game of grab-ass with an adult Harry Potter.

Later, I found Woody staggering around the bar, trying to hold up a giant glass boot full of beer. He gave me a hug, sloshing the contents of the boot down my back, and called me a fucker. I helped him onto a table after he insisted he wanted to dance a jig.

After that tournament, I became a permanent member of the team and usually the first sub in as a spark plug, which says a lot about my skill…or shows there is a very shallow player pool. Over the next eight years, I traveled to eight countries, representing the

U.S. on the Paralympic team while so much of my life unfolded: my comedy career exploded, and I got married and had a son. But I'm getting ahead of myself, gentle reader.

◯)◯)◯)

Once I established myself on the team, I joined the cool kids' table with the team captain Josh McKinney. McKinney is shy and soft-spoken; he's damn near a mute. He became my best friend on the team, and we bunked together as often as we could. That may not have been a good thing. I'm probably the reason we never won another tournament, because I would keep our star player up, giggling long into the night. One time, I jokingly told him I put my balls on his pillow, and no matter how many times I assured him I was joking, he was up late grappling with the thought. He couldn't sleep at all, and the next day he played like shit. At least he never told Coach Moss the source of his insomnia.

On our trip to Russia, we stayed in a children's dormitory outside Moscow. McKinney and I roomed together, and on our first day, our new athletic trainer walked by our open door.

"Hey Brad, can you come in here?" McKinney yelled.

Brad stood in the doorway, expecting us to ask for help taping our ankles or stretching our calves.

"Can you help us push our beds together?" I asked with my straightest of faces. Seeing the look of bewilderment on his face, I continued. "Yeah, we play better if we can touch when we sleep." He made two hesitant steps forward before McKinney and I cracked, bursting into laughter.

The team was in Argentina for the Pan-American games. It was my third tournament, and I had established my position on the team. I was a competitive player with a sharp tongue and even sharper elbows. None of this was contributing to any success on the field. Our team was losing games eight to nil. I couldn't seem to duplicate my breakout success from the EuroCup, no matter what I did.

I've never had the endurance to be a starter and play a whole game. I thought practice was the little soccer activities I was already doing. I would bring my ball everywhere, especially when I was on the road for comedy. I would kick it around the hotel room: lamps for twenty points, televisions for ten. I would bring the ball to the club and warm up in the lobby, juggling it and passing it to unwilling fans before my shows, to the dismay of the club owner. I wish I had tried harder for my team's sake, and because of the fact that I was representing my country. I truly loved playing the game.

I've always had a high metabolism, but when I played soccer, I was ravenous; I could never get full or hydrated. My stomach could be sloshing full of Powerade, and I would still be pissing dehydrated yellow. I had a stash of granola bars and gummy bears, and a barrel full of Powerade next to my bed. I woke up three times a night like a groggy bear coming out of hibernation to eat. Many nights McKinney would wake up to find me on the edge of my bed, half-naked, mouth smacking full of gummy bears, staring at him dead-eyed. Breakfast could never come soon enough.

Every country we played in had its unique twist on breakfast: Russia had borscht and greasy, grenade-shaped sausages; Argentina had green eggs and ham; Brazil had all the exotic fruits you could imagine; Holland had ham and cheese for breakfast, lunch, and dinner.

This particular morning in Argentina I was so hungry, and my stomach was going full Karen. I was in the long buffet line with McCullough, piling little Vienna sausages on my plate. These were the kind that didn't have rounded edges, just two-inch long tubes that look like they'd been cut out of the same infinitely long sausage. Too hungry to wait, I popped one of the greasy little tubes in my mouth. Fighting its impending doom, it decided to escape and squirted back out like a lubed legless hamster. McCullough was reaching for the sausages just as the projectile landed back into the giant pan of its buddies and disappeared. John dropped the sausage scoop. We looked at each other with wild eyes and slid our trays onward to the egg pan.

We were traveling around the world, but we didn't have much time to explore on our own. When we weren't practicing or playing, the coaches wanted us to rest. There were a few planned sight-seeing trips for the team in every country.

In Brazil, we saw a soccer game between two rival pro teams at Maracana Stadium, the largest in Brazil and the biggest one I'd ever seen. The atmosphere inside was absolute mayhem. People brought little grills and were cooking at their feet. When the home team scored, fans would throw what seemed like sticks of dynamite onto the field. The visiting team's supporters were secured in an area that resembled a prison, with high fences and armed guards so the home fans couldn't rip them apart. At the end of the game, these fans were escorted out of the stadium by a column of marching police in full riot gear on horseback, wielding six-foot wooden batons.

In Chile, we attended a pro soccer game with a unique halftime tradition where the referees and linesmen ran as fast as they could to center field accompanied by riot police with shields.

The crowd would then jeer and yell insults and rain down glass bottles upon them. It seemed very cathartic—and fun—for everyone involved.

In Russia there were no soccer games for us to visit, so we saw Red Square and Stalin's grave instead. They housed us in a seemingly abandoned Jewish primary school that had no hot water, and the ice cold water we did get came out in a thin trickle. Every time someone took a shower, we all knew because of the agonizing screams. I befriended the school groundskeeper despite our language barrier, and we laughed over his secret stash of vodka.

In every country we got to go shopping in their outdoor markets. During our trip to Chile, we were weeble-wobbling through a bustling open-air market; twelve disabled Americans guarding their backpacks and wallets against pickpockets, and painfully aware of how conspicuous we were.

McCullough pointed out, "Hey Bluey, why you always have this pack of dogs following you?"

"What do you mean?" I looked around to find seven dogs trailing me.

"I noticed that everywhere we go, there's at least one dog tailing you."

It was a busy market, but they were clearly following me. My response was some mumblings about Africa. Until then, I hadn't thought it was strange. After that, I took note, and sure enough, most everywhere I went, there was some stray dog following me like I was the alpha. There were a couple occasions when people went as far as to ask me, "Hey mister, what's your dog's name?"

Perhaps they were following me because of the day I infiltrated the sleeping pack in Africa. Or maybe they were simply following the person who had the potential for making the most crumbs and had the lingering odor of sausage. I'm surprised none of those dogs ever made it onto the field.

Eventually, our beloved coach Rick Moss was replaced with Jay Hoffman, a real hard-ass. He was a stickler for fitness, and he demanded we compete at a higher level. He came over from the U.S. Women's Olympic team, where he had been the assistant coach on one of the best soccer squads ever. He had experience working with top-of-the-line athletes like Mia Hamm, but now he was with us, or more specifically, with my lazy cherry-pickin' ass.

There were soccer camps peppered throughout the year, usually at the Olympic training center in Chula Vista, California. I attended as many of them as my burgeoning comedy tour schedule would permit. It was a balancing act between two worlds I truly loved, comedy and soccer, but I was a starter in comedy and a backup on the Paralympic team. For a lot of people, being on that team was the most important thing in their lives and their legacy, but for me, it ended up more of a side gig, and it showed in my fitness. I probably could have been a starter if I put in the work, but I would rather drink and smoke weed after a show than do crunches or wind sprints. I realized as we went along that there were enough camps to make me feel like it was real, but not enough to make me feel like we could win a medal.

What we were up against slowly came into focus. The four world powerhouses were Russia, Ukraine, Brazil, and Iran. They all had their own living and training facilities, and practiced twice a day year-round. They were cohesive units on the pitch, and it showed when they played. Some of the players were so good, it was hard to determine what their disability was, or if they even had one. When we played them, we knew it would be the longest sixty minutes of our lives, both physically and mentally, and we had to pick the ball out of the back of our net at least ten times. Some of the guys on my team were still learning the fundamentals, because, like me, they never had the chance to play on a team in their formative years. Against athletes of this caliber, in most games I felt like a spectator on the field—best seat in the house, at least until after the game when Coach Hoffman chewed you out and gave you some extra laps.

I was experiencing a strange convergence of successes in my careers. I was at the top of my disability class, playing on the world's stage for my country's national team. When I wasn't hanging with top players on the pitch, I was hanging with top players on the comedy stage. I was making the headliners work. Some famous comics had complained to the club that they didn't want me opening for them anymore because I was damn near impossible to follow. To realize you have that power over these big names is eye-opening. Winning on the stage gave me the fortitude to go back and lose on the pitch.

()()()

Soccer is a beautiful way to express yourself. It's a thinking man's game. If I can fight through palsy elbows and kick the ball to where I anticipate you're going, and you score a goal, it's like playing a multi-level chess game in the bed of a pickup truck barreling down a dirt road. When you strike the ball—just right—there's no better feeling than when it comes off your foot and goes where you intended it to. The amazing thing about soccer is everyone has their own unique style of play, but, when on a team, they have to become a cohesive unit. The ultimate team chemistry is one that's predictable to your teammates and unpredictable to your opponents. You can be the best player in the world, but if no one can get you the ball, what's the point? Every Messi has his Di María.

The Paralympics were subject to the same stringent drug testing as the able-bodied Olympics. The anti-doping agency would randomly come to an athlete's house to test them for prohibited substances. If you weren't there, they called your cell phone, and you had one hour to get back. If not, you were marked as a no-show. You were allowed three no-shows before you were kicked off your prospective team. Every athlete filled out a monthly form, identifying times and places where they would be. For most athletes, this was an inconvenience. For me, it was damn near impossible. Most athletes have a pretty regular routine, like "I'll be in the gym, Monday, Wednesday, and Friday." Trying to tell them my schedule was crazy: "I'll be in Nebraska Monday, Idaho Wednesday, and New York Friday."

Drug testing is a scary endeavor, especially when you're a comedian. My comedy and soccer lifestyles were juxtaposed against each other. One was about staying up late and partying with your peers, the other was about getting up early and pushing your body to the limit. Soccer was testing to make sure I didn't have illegal substances in my system, and comedy was about keeping those very substances fresh in my body.

The first time I was drug tested at home, I was rudely jostled awake from sleeping off a hangover by an insistent, authoritative knock on my door. It was 7 a.m. on the dot. I staggered out in my boxers and cracked the door open to find two large Black men in matching business casual.

"Hello, we're looking for Josh Blue," the smaller of the two said.

"He may be here. It depends on who's asking," I replied, clearly matching the photo on their clipboard.

"We are with the United States Anti-Doping Agency, and we're here to collect a urine sample."

"Okay, let me get him," I said and let them in the front door.

They watched through my bedroom door as I sniff-checked my t-shirts for the one that smelled the least skunky. I threw on shorts and said a prayer. I knew I hadn't done any soccer performance-enhancing drugs, but I'd definitely smoked a lot of weed that week. And the five years before that.

I came out and offered them a seat and a breakfast beer. They introduced themselves as what I remember to be Gigantor and Gigantor Jr. While Junior sat on my couch, Gigantor opted to stand and make me feel nervous. The man on the couch gestured for me to come sit next to him as he explained how the process worked.

"You'll pick one of these five sterile, sealed containers. After you open the package, we'll make sure the numbers on the box match the two jars inside. Once you're done with that, you'll go into the bathroom with Gigantor, and you'll need to pull your shirt up to your nipples and your shorts down to your knees. He will need to have a clear view of the urine leaving your body. Once we've entered your home and identified it's you, you're not allowed to leave our sight."

As he was talking, I was power chugging water and looking around, trying to decide the best window to jump out of.

"Once the cup is full, you will come back out here and put it on your coffee table," he gestured to the table in front of us covered with a pipe, rolling papers, and weed crumbs.

In the bathroom, I attempted small talk as I pulled shirt to nipples and shorts to knees; one of the more awkward positions I've ever been in. Peeing in a cup is no easy task; I have trouble getting it in the toilet under the best of circumstances. I knew holding the cup would be a disaster. Standing there, middle-half-naked, I asked Gigantor if it was okay if I put the cup in the sink and tried to pee into it like a carnival game.

"If that's what you have to do, boss." He gave off a real John Coffey vibe from *The Green Mile*.

This created a more awkward situation for me, because the sink was a little higher, so I had to stand on tiptoe, with my balls on the cold porcelain, and try to not focus on the fact that there was a large man standing behind me. I had more stage fright peeing in front of one person than I did performing in front of thousands of people on a real stage. Every time I was about to release, I would look in the medicine cabinet mirror and see Gigantor standing two heads taller than me, arms crossed, making the pee crawl back up. I tried to lighten the mood, but he was a tough audience.

"I've been working on my glutes. What do you think?"

Silence.

I kept chugging water, and it took forever for my bladder to fill up enough to release, despite having someone eagerly awaiting my pee's arrival. The whole ordeal took about fifteen minutes, but it feels like I'm still waiting to go. When the dam finally broke, the stream was strong enough to knock over the unsuspecting cup. I frantically righted it, pissing on my own hand, and began to rapidly fill it, realizing there was enough for five cups.

Once I stopped, the man told me to screw the lid on tight.

"Can I pull up my shorts first?" I asked.

Putting the cover on was nerve-wracking. More pee sloshed out on my hands. Just another morning in the Josh Blue abode. But I was able to capture enough for the sample.

Back on the couch, Gigantor Jr. pretended like it hadn't taken forever. "Now I need you to pour the pee into these two sterile, sealed containers."

I told him that would not be possible, and he would have to do it.

"That would be against protocol. Each athlete needs to be in charge of their own urine."

"That ain't gonna happen, bro. Liquids and me aren't compatible."

After a moment where Gigantor shared a look with Junior that told him the bathroom was now a piss Slip 'N Slide, he relented.

"Okay, I see this is a special circumstance. I can do it, but I will need to write a detailed report of what I did."

"Whatever you gotta do," I said. "I just don't want pee all over my living room."

Once that was done, he boxed everything up, and they shook my pee hand with great reluctance. I lied and said it was a pleasure to meet them as I escorted them to the door, feeling somewhat violated.

The weeks between the test and the results, I felt a heavy, impending doom. Would I be kicked off the team for marijuana use? It was an immense relief when the test came back negative, but they must have detected the marijuana, because I was "randomly" tested a lot more than anyone else on my team. It was always those same two guys. I guess they liked the show.

After my curious passing grade, I found out there are two types of testing: in-competition and out-of-competition. When you are out-of-competition you can have cannabinoids in your system. From then on, a month out from any competition, I would stop smoking weed.

I learned so much about the anti-doping agency, and doping doesn't always come in the form of drugs. I learned that before a wheelchair race, the judges inspect a paralyzed athlete's body to make sure they have not stuck any nails into their legs. Athletes do this because they can't feel it, but the body recognizes the foreign object and kicks up the adrenaline. *Ah, man. We're definitely going to lose. I'm not that dedicated to this.* I'd be the guy at the start of the race, like "Aw fuck, I forgot my nail!"

I was in Rio de Janeiro, Brazil, on Copacabana Beach with my teammates. Coach Hoffman had surprised us by scrapping practice and letting us go to the beach for a recovery day to rejuvenate our muscles in the frigid ocean. The no practice thing was a new side of our coach. He was a stickler for routine. My teammate Tommy Latch and I were playing catch with a football in the surf. I had brought an American football to toss around in downtime, but more importantly, to test the coaches' patience.

The day before, I was on this same section of beach with Tommy under completely different conditions. It was cold and the rain blew sideways. Tommy and I were the only ones dumb enough to be out in the storm. The ocean churned and the waves collided at random angles. The ocean was pissed off that day, and I didn't want to turn my back on it. We were playing catch and goofing around when a withered old man turned up out of the rain. When he saw a couple of disabled guys with only two good arms between them, he slowed his pace. My arm is bad, but Tommy's looks like a deep-fried chicken wing, plus or minus the barbecue sauce, depending on what he ate that day. The old man scolded us in Portuguese and frantically gestured for us to come onto shore.

"We're only knee-deep," I said, laughing to Tommy indignantly, and we waved the old man off.

Today was completely different. The white sand reflected the bright sun, and the beach was heavily dotted with beautiful Brazilian women in tiny swimsuits and men in swimsuits the same size. The waves were heavy and crashing, but the sun made them seem less ominous.

We were thigh-deep in the water when a big wave came in. I could tell by the way the wave hit Tommy how strong it was—his body jerked, and the water crashed up around his chest. He dove under, and I followed. When we came up, it was like somebody had pulled the plug in the ocean.

What was a playful surf a moment before had turned into an uncontrollable force of water, indifferently pulling me away from shore. As I dug in and tried to stand my ground, I felt little rocks and sharp shells rushing past my legs, bouncing off my shins. It felt like I was on a treadmill on a level that was way out of my league. In half a second, I was sucked out with all those little shells; we put up the same amount of resistance to the power of the ocean. The only difference was that those little shells lived underwater.

By the time the water stopped pulling, I was chest-deep and in awe, my brain racing to figure out how to get to shore. I looked over and saw Tommy, the same distance out but twenty yards to my right. He looked surprised but was doing a good job of treading water with his chicken wing. Five feet from Tommy, there was a young couple who were doing all right for themselves, but when they saw me floundering, they shook their heads to say, *sorry, you're on your own.*

This was the kind of water that would throw around a good swimmer, and I'm not what you could even reasonably call a swimmer. The next wave passed over my head, and I struggled to get on top of it, hoping for a ride back to shore, but the undertow dragged me deeper. I flashed back to a third grade Special Ed swim class and the teacher telling us, "If you ever get in a scary situation, just remain calm."

"Heeelp!" I shrieked, my head barely above water.

My calm evaporated, and I knew I wasn't getting out of this by myself. My heart jackhammered in my chest, and my muscles burned from struggling to keep me alive. All those missed fitness opportunities were coming back to haunt me.

People on the beach started to take notice. The ones who didn't know me looked more concerned than my teammates. They probably figured, "That's just Bluey, jack-assin' around." I was the Boy Who Cried Comedy.

By the time the third wave crashed over me, everybody knew I needed help. I opened my eyes with a good four feet of water above me, and I could see lightning bolt sunbeams refracting down. I thought about my pregnant wife back home, grateful that I had at least passed on some of the Blue lineage before my imminent doom. Thinking about my unborn son, I pushed off the sandy bottom and broke through the surface, my burning eyes wild with desperation.

People were gathering on the beach. Finally, a hero jumped in. He had Honey-Nut Cheerios hair and a beach bum tan.

Just remain calm.

Every time I was forced under, I'd gulp big mouthfuls of sandy, salty seawater. When I clawed back to the surface, I'd suck air in such a panic that I was hyperventilating. There was always another wave coming that could end me.

By the time the guy got to me, I was almost resigned to let the next wave take me. *If he's not here by the time the next wave comes, I'm just going to give up.*

"Don't fight it!" the guy yelled. "Swim with the current!"

"I'm not fucking swimming, sir!" Even at death's door, I was able to splutter a joke.

"I am going to help you," he said with an angelic accent. He was treading water, offering me his elbow. I realized he was apprehensive about helping me. He knew the desperation of the situation. As panicked as I was, I could have dragged him down with me. I remembered another lesson from that distant swim class: *If you're drowning, stay calm and let them help you.*

The guy stopped just out of reach, treading water and assessing if I could be helped without putting himself in more danger. Was I too panicked for him to risk it? I worried he might swim away at any moment.

"I'm going to help you steady yourself."

He offered me his arm, but I didn't hook into his elbow. I pressed my hand against him to steady myself. It wasn't until I saw Freezer, the Paralympic athletic trainer, swimming toward us that I started to feel better. Not good, but at least I knew they would recover my body. Freezer was a triathlete. I was hoping one of his three disciplines was saving drowning cripples.

When Freezer got up close, he offered me an elbow like the beach bum had, and again, I pressed against him just enough to stabilize myself. I had the other guy's elbow with my left hand, and as soon as I touched Freezer, I had a sense I was going to make it through this, though I couldn't catch my breath. As soon as I had that thought, another wave crashed over me, and when I resurfaced, I was no longer holding onto them. They were holding onto me. I'm not certain how many more waves I swallowed before they dragged me to shore.

The next thing I remember, we were where Tommy and I had started before we got sucked out, in ankle deep water. The sun reflected more brilliantly off the yellow sand, and everybody's bathing suits popped out in vivid colors. I could see myself from above being pulled out of the water, the tops of my feet being dragged over the sharp coral on the beach, my two saviors Freezer and Beach Bum holding me by the armpits. I remember people gawking at me, slack-jawed, pointing and asking, "Is he dead?" I could feel the sand scraping against my feet, but I could also see those feet. They were blue, and my hands were blue, too. As blue as my name.

I couldn't regulate my breath, and my heart was pounding in my head. It felt like I had just sprinted my fastest for seven miles. My lungs were out of control, painfully trying to refill my body with oxygen.

They dragged me up to the dry sand. It was delightfully hot and dry. I remember thinking, *I can't believe I'm still alive*. But also thinking, *I don't know if I'm out of this yet*. I was breathing too hard, and I felt like I'd never catch my breath again. They put me down as gently as they could, which wasn't very gentle because they were themselves exhausted. I was lying on my side. My head lay on the deliciously warm sand. Just as my breathing started to slow, the puking began.

The first paramedic on the scene was a stout, barefoot, barrel-chested man in no particular hurry. The second paramedic was barefoot too, but I remembered the stout guy, because he was the one who did the talking. They wanted to take me to the hospital, but I tried to wave them away, finally managing to gasp, "How much is it going to cost me?" I didn't have insurance, and I didn't think I could afford it.

"It's free," they said. They insisted. They thought I might have sand in my lungs. They weren't about to leave me there.

I hesitantly agreed, and they loaded me on the stretcher in nothing but my swimsuit, and carried me to the ambulance. My breathing had almost returned to normal, and now my biggest worry was the staring. My teammates walked alongside the stretcher, concerned, hollering encouragement.

"Don't die, Bluey!"

"We need you on the pitch!"

Tommy put my football back into my arms, and I was relieved to see he had escaped the ocean. A teammate named Louis piped up, "I wanted to throw that to you while you were drowning, you could have put it under your chin like a life preserver."

The locals didn't even stop their sand soccer game, as if they had seen people drown on that beach every day.

The paramedics lifted me into the back of the ambulance, and Freezer climbed in after us. He spent the ride trying to communicate with the paramedics. I listened blankly. Their poor English was no match for our shitty Portuguese. There was a rectangular window above my head; I saw all the trees with their vibrant flowers in bloom. I saw the beautiful sunny sky with white rolling clouds. And then, right into that frame, came the image of Christ the Redeemer, the giant statue of Jesus with his arms stretched out in welcome. You don't get a better view of Brazil than from a stretcher in the back of an ambulance. I pointed at the statue and called out to Freezer. He looked out, put his hand on my arm, and said, "Yeah. He's the reason you're here today."

"No," I told him. "You're the reason I'm here."

"He's the one that gave me the strength to do what I had to do," he said.

"No," I said. "You're a triathlete."

Upon arrival at the ER my heart rate felt close to normal, and I had control over my breathing. I was met with a wheelchair. I said I could walk, but they said it wasn't optional.

"You don't have any shoes on."

Soon I was grateful for their insistence. The floor of the hospital was like a Jackson Pollock canvas splattered with mud, debris, and blood, both fresh and dry. It was chaos in the waiting room: people in bandages, people moaning, stab wounds, dog bites, babies screaming, shouting, doctors and nurses slip-sliding down the hallway. It was all the mayhem of an American ER minus the sanitary precautions.

Freezer tried to help me with the paperwork. My needs were not urgent compared to gun shots and monkey bites, so I waited for quite some time before they finally got me to the x-ray room. After they x-rayed my torso, they told me the doctor would see me shortly, and then parked my wheelchair in the hallway next to an old woman who seemed peacefully dead on her gurney with her hands folded on her chest. I was starting to feel like the hospital experience was more traumatic than the near-drowning. For the next hour I studied her body for any signs of life, which were apparently not present.

They wheeled me into a large, open examination room with several hospital beds. It was as chaotic in there as it was out in the hall. Someone assured me that the doctor would look at my x-ray momentarily, then the door burst open. A middle-aged woman ran in clasping her throat, making the most terrifying gurgling noises. She was having an allergic reaction, and her throat was closing, producing mass amounts of saliva which was streaming from her mouth. Her eyes were bulging from her head while everyone was trying to corral her to a bed. For some reason she started spinning in circles, her arms out to the side and saliva flying out of her like a sprinkler system.

I looked at Freezer. "I'm fine. I'd like to go back to the hotel now."

It turns out, I was fine.

It took three days to fully recover from "recovery day." Every joint in my body creaked and crackled with all the salt in my system. It felt like I had malaria again.

Back at the hotel, my teammates tentatively came to my room one by one to check on me. Later, McKinney arrived with some dinner. He informed me someone had actually drowned that day, not too far from where they dragged me in.

"All the other teams think it was you," he said. "Just now at dinner a delegate from each team came and gave me condolences."

"Did you tell them I was still alive?" I asked.

"No," he said. "We need every advantage we can get in this tournament."

()()()

In 2004, we barely qualified for the summer Paralympics in Athens, Greece. But we did it! What a trip, mentally and physically. Somehow, in my limited time playing the sport I love, I made it to the highest point you can reach in a Paralympic career. The Paralympics is the second largest sporting event on the planet. And the fact it was being held in Athens, the birthplace of the modern Olympic Games, back in 1896, blew my mind.

The U.S. delegation chartered a flight from D.C. to Greece. Every team sport was there, from wheelchair basketball to the notoriously mischievous bocce ball boys. It took four hours for everyone to load onto the jumbo jet. I was convinced that of all the flights I had been on, this was the flight that was going to crash. Just what the news cycle needed: "In other weird news, hundreds of America's top crippled athletes went to their watery grave in the Atlantic. They were so…inspirational. They died doing what they loved—drowning. Back to you, Diane."

After unloading the plane and boarding the buses, it had already been a very long day. Athens hadn't remodeled since the last Olympics; the Parthenon and the Acropolis were all run down.

The gates at the Olympic Village were guarded by machine-gun-wielding military men, and the enormity of the event started to sink in. The able-bodied Olympics had been held there two weeks prior, and we would be staying in the same facilities. The U.S. being one of the largest delegations, there were four 12-story buildings that housed us. By comparison, a smaller country like Togo would have only one or two rooms.

We had a few days to get acclimated before the Paralympics got started. I was ready to play. We tried to find activities that didn't consume too much energy, even though my adrenaline was racing in anticipation of the ass whooping we were about to receive. Each floor in the dorms had its own balcony. After dinner, most of the athletes would gather on their respective balconies and yell across to each other. The U.S. women's wheelchair basketball team was directly across from us, and we flirted from afar.

The night before the opening ceremonies, we were all out on our balconies, enjoying the cool breeze, when down the road we could hear the bocce ball boys shouting in an unintelligible palsy fury. We turned to see both of them going full-throttle in their souped-up power wheelchairs, one chasing the other. As they got closer, cheers started to rise from the balconies. The guy in front had a devilish smile, I dubbed him the Instigator. The chaser had murder in his eyes, giggling like a psycho. He had to be the Giggler.

As they zoomed up the road and between the dorms, all the delegations had picked their sides and were cheering for their favorite. The Instigator made a mistake getting his wheelchair wedged too close to the curb, ending up with nowhere to go. He was violently slammed from behind by the Giggler, which caused him to laugh so contagiously that all the spectators in this coliseum-like scenario were soon roaring along as his teammate attempted to kill him.

The Instigator freed his wheelchair and turned to face his foe. A series of unintelligible words came from both sides as they circled each other like two feral cats in an alley. Then someone from one of the upper floors finally yelled it: "Cripple fiiight!" It was echoed throughout the entire Olympic Village.

"Cripple fiiight!"

"Cripple fiiight!"

This was a reference from the devastating *South Park* episode I had watched with my friends back in college. But now I was surrounded by hundreds of my fellow disabled people not only owning it but also chanting it in unison. The bocce boys, needing no encouragement, accelerated toward one another and collided, tangling themselves in a blur of flailing appendages and shrieking sounds only a palsy throat could produce. They broke apart and circled each other again in their power chairs. The Giggler issued a new challenge, and it was on. To our surprise they both slithered out of their wheelchairs and squirmed across the hot blacktop until they were in striking distance. They hit each other with any part of their body that worked and some that didn't. By this time, the audience's cheers and exhausted laughter were at a fevered pitch. We were supposed to be taking it easy in preparation for the games, but we all got a heavy ab workout.

Their coach dutifully trudged out and peeled the boys apart, scolding all of us for egging them on. You can keep your UFC, this was the bout of the century. I'd pay top dollar to see it again. The boys triumphantly dragged themselves back to their wheelchairs, clearly enjoying the spotlight. Watching them fight their way up into the seats seemed like more of a battle than the epic duel they had just fought. The Paralympics hadn't even started, but we all got a free preview of how thrilling disabled sport can be.

The next day, as we prepared to enter the arena for the opening ceremonies, Coach Hoffman called us all to attention.

"I'd like to remind you boys that you are representing your country. And I don't wanna hear nothin' about no kind of 'cripple fights.' And if I hear that yelled by any one of you, I'll send you home on the next plane, because there are plenty of other boys who would be more than happy to take your spot."

All my teammates looked at me. If anyone was going to get sent home for having fun, I was the guy.

The opening ceremony was a giant game of hurry up and wait. The logistics of organizing 135 participating countries with 3,806 athletes, each with their own unique disability, was the definition of a clusterfuck. It took them almost four and a half hours before they got to the U.S., and I was half-asleep on my feet when they called Uganda. Instead of tempting fate by yelling "cripple fight," I tempted fate a different way by flirting with a woman named Patty from the wheelchair basketball team. By the time the United States was introduced, I was more into her than the spectacle surrounding us. She was a fiery Latina, paralyzed from the waist down, with a raspy voice that could rip the paint off a wagon.

All in all, the opening ceremony took damn near nine hours. My parents flew in from Minnesota to support me, and my college roommate Togashi flew in from Japan. I guess it was a pretty big event, 1.6 billion people worldwide watched it, but unfortunately, none of them were in the United States. It was quite a controversy; no American network stayed after the able-bodied Olympics to broadcast the event. This lack of coverage was why I hadn't heard of the Paralympics until my fellow counselor at Easter Seals had clued me in. In the twenty years since, American media has made slow but steady progress in supporting disabled sports.

Back at the Olympic Village, it was more hurry up and wait. There were a few recreational buildings set up around the Village with ping-pong, pool, and some video games. They were places you could go without your countrymen and meet people from all over the world. I was disappointed to find there was no Cameroonian delegation, but I did find the Senegalese, and I sought out the other French-speaking nations.

My favorite place to people watch was the cafeteria, a giant structure with row upon row of lunch tables, food from all over the world, and thousands of disabled people, not just surviving, but thriving. What a beautiful ordeal. Every variation on every disability. One of my favorite things was the wheelchair trains. Someone in a big power chair was the engine, and there were seven or eight push chairs in a chain, latched onto the one in front of them, lunch trays in their laps.

I had one of those rare moments—I felt like I truly belonged. There were varying degrees of disability, but we were all on the same uneven playing field. No one was being zeroed in on. If there's one disabled person in the room, everyone stares at us. In the cafeteria, there were so many disabled people to stare at, nobody knew *who* to stare at.

It was two days before everyone started staring at me again. I'd walk in with my teammates and say, "Hey why is everyone looking at me? For fuck's sake there's a guy over there eating with his foot!"

Am I just loud and obnoxious? For whatever reason, they definitely were gawking at me. I'd like to say it was my devilish good looks, but probably…loud and obnoxious.

Over the next couple weeks, I would occasionally take Patty to the cafeteria for a cheap date, a.k.a. free meal. We'd laugh and flirt, and say horrible things. One day over frozen yogurt, I was sitting across from her at one of the lunch tables. After a while I said to her, "Patty, I've been playing footsie with you for the last forty minutes."

"I'm paralyzed from the waist down. I can't feel my legs, you dumbass!"

"Oh, I thought you were just stone cold, 'cause my foot was like halfway up your thigh."

There were eight seven-a-side football teams in the 2004 Summer Paralympics. Spoiler alert: we came in eighth. There were two round-robins, and the one we were in was the more difficult of the two. Our first game—against Russia—we lost 3-0. The Russian team was phenomenal. Some of their players were so good, after a little while I was like, "There's nothing even fucking wrong with that guy." I wanted to wave the ref over and say, "Hey man, I call bullshit on number five. Get a neurologist out here." Then number five would run by, and I'd be like, "Aw shit, never mind, his hand is on backward."

Next, we lost to Brazil 4-0. It was a hard-fought game, but they had that beautiful sport etched in their souls. They grew up playing it, and they just wanted it more. They were so good, I wanted to check their legs for nails.

By the time we lost our second game, we knew we weren't advancing, and the other athletes stopped asking us how our games went. Soccer is an international language most of the United States does not speak. The rest of the world looked at us like the runty kid that was up to bat: "Easy out!"

Our third and final match was against Holland. We lost 6-1. The silver lining was that we didn't get completely shut out. Brazil and Russia advanced, and Argentina and Ukraine moved forward from the other group. We were out, and we had a week and a half before the closing ceremony. Our days were filled with hard practices. Coach took his disappointment and frustration out on us through fitness, with practices that didn't involve a soccer ball.

"You think the Ruskies get tired?" he would yell as he continued to run our already broken bodies into the ground.

When Brazil played Argentina, it was a complete and utter bloodbath. The two teams were notorious for their dirty play. I know from personal experience; I received quite a few elbows to the ribs and cleats raked across the Achilles. The game got more intense as it went on; we could feel the simmering tension between the two teams, and somewhere in the second half there was a bench-clearing brawl. It wasn't just fourteen guys on the field fighting, it was all the backups mixed with the athletic trainers, coaches, and staff. It was complete mayhem. Some players were chasing each other, some players were squared off trading blows, and if I were to do commentary on the fight: "The Brazilian throws a left, and another left, and another left, and another left! That five-six just beat up a seven!" If the bocce boys had a cripple fight, this was world war cripple. The violence went on forever, and the crowd was booing. It was a disgrace to the spirit of the Olympics. After at least ten minutes the referees finally restored order and ejected nine players, leaving three Argentinians and two Brazilians to finish the game. *I bet we could take Brazil now*. The final score was 4-1 Brazil.

Then there was the Russia vs. Ukraine game. The best soccer match I've ever seen. It was one of those hard-fought games that looked like they were playing for something more than a win. There was no bench-clearing brawl, but they played with the highest intensity. Ukraine ended up beating Russia 4-1. I would soon discover what that loss would mean to the Russian players.

That night in the cafeteria, the Russian coach walked in, leading a solemn, single file line of his losing players. They walked in unison, like a column of soldiers. The coach led them to the chow line. He got himself a tray and proceeded to heap food onto it. All the players followed him, but none of them picked up a tray. He led them to an empty table where he sat at the head while we watched him mechanically eat this giant mound of food. I kind of hated the Russians before this; now I just felt bad for them. Losing in their country means you don't get to eat.

We lost all three of our games by a margin of 13-1, and I was gleefully gobbling down my second cheeseburger. Sure we had done some extra running as punishment, but at least we got our supper.

Word had spread that I was a stand-up comedian, and more and more people started asking me to do a show for the U.S. delegation. The thought of it excited and terrified me. It would be my first international show and the first for an audience entirely of people with disabilities. These are the people I'm giving voice to, the people I'm making fun of.

Two days before the closing ceremonies, a good portion of the delegation gathered in the basement of one of our dorms. The majority of people were done competing in their events, but there was still a handful of Olympic hopefuls in the audience. I paced outside, feeling nauseous and needing to pee. At this point I was only two years into my comedy career and still a relative rookie. I didn't want to bomb, especially after our dismal performance on the field. I don't think anyone introduced me. I awkwardly picked my way to the middle of the room through the wheelchairs, crutches, and braces, up to the shitty mic, and the rest was a blur. Theater in the round. With wild gestures, twisting and turning, playing to everyone in the audience, and getting tangled in the meager four feet of cable that anchored me to the spot, I scraped through twenty-seven of the thirty minutes I had planned to do.

I was super nervous to see how my peers would react to my jokes about my disability. The majority laughed at the right parts, but my teammates laughed the hardest, especially at the parts no one else laughed at, which is what good friends do. Everyone applauded at the end, at least the ones who were capable.

The soccer boys and I went to root for Patty and the Women's Wheelchair National Basketball team in their gold medal game. They had all the fight we did not, all the way up to their gold medal win. After the game, in basketball tradition, each woman on the U.S. team took a turn climbing a ladder to cut the net off the hoop.

Yes, you read that right. These women from the wheelchair basketball team climbed a ladder to cut the net. Watching these women fight their way up this ladder made me embarrassed about the effort we had put forth. Instead of saying that, I turned to my teammates. "You thought winning Olympic gold was hard, try climbing a ladder with dead legs."

"Dammit, Bluey."

Throughout the closing ceremony, I held hands with Patty, while she teased me about not having a medal. I had mixed feelings about going home. I was ready to get back to the comedy life, but I also wanted to hang out with Patty more. I missed the limelight of stand-up. Even if we had won a gold medal, nobody back home would know about it, let alone care. You can't care about something you don't even know exists.

Uninformed Americans mix up the Special Olympics with the Paralympics. This symbolizes a greater problem: People don't recognize the difference between a mental disability and a physical disability. In other countries, they embrace the Paralympics, and people do care. Their athletes have a chance to return home as heroes, not simply as disabled.

As for Patty, we dated for a few months, and she accidentally introduced me to my future ex-wife. So really, a total loss all around on the 2004 Paralympics.

240 | *Something To Stare At*

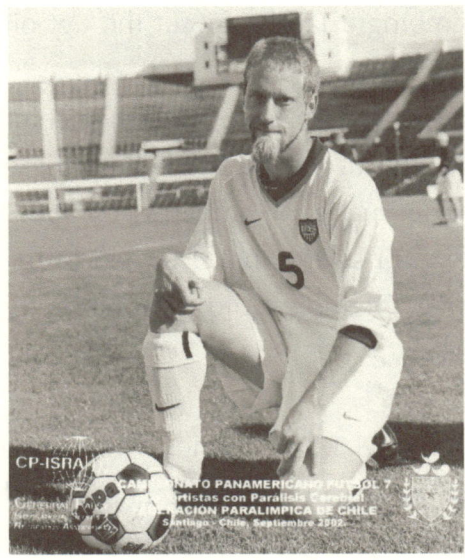

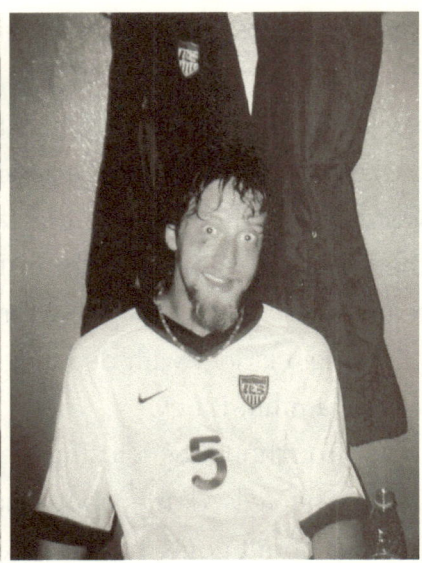

Me before and after any given game.

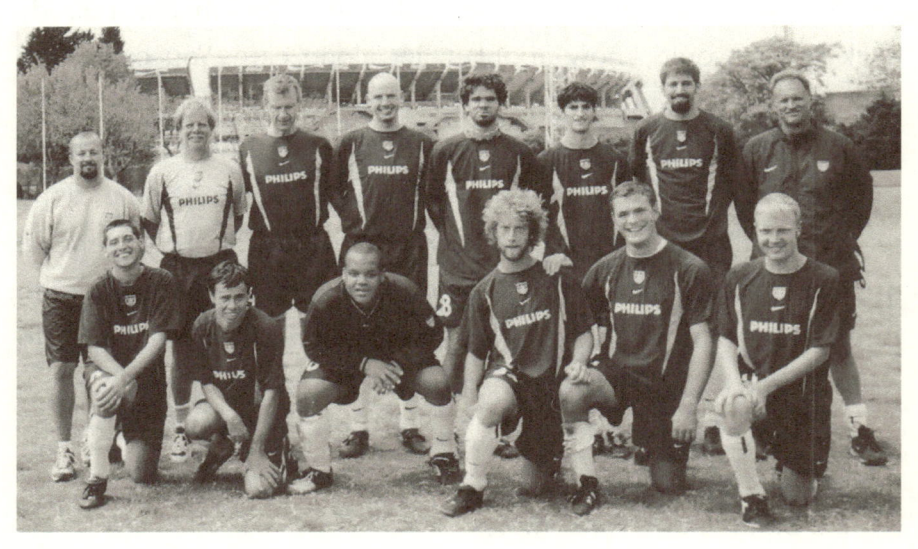

The 2003 U.S. Men's Paralympic Soccer Team. Clockwise from left: Team Trainer Brad, Hardass Coach Jay Hoffman, John Theobald The Yeller, Jon McCullough aka Mr. Clean, Hall of Famer Joshua McKinney, Smartass Eli Wolff, Captain Michael Peters, Assistant Coach Michael Haas aka Coach Numble Nuts, Jason Slemons aka Slammer, Roman Grier the Southern Belle, Bluey, Keith Johnson aka Muck, David Woosnam aka Wobbly Woozy, Tom Latsch aka Chicken Wing.

COMEDY ACT II

After two years of performing comedy, I'd come to know the Comedy Works club and the local scene, but I was ignorant of the stand-up world outside of Denver. My more experienced peers saw the trajectory I was on and encouraged me to find management.

It turned out that Comedy Works had a separate management company called Comedy Works Entertainment, run by a guy named Mike Raftery. His office was located right above the downtown club, so on a random Wednesday, I mustered enough courage to go find him. Not sure of the proper etiquette when shopping for a manager, I entered the office and tossed a poorly recorded VHS tape from a Raschke room performance on his desk. "Hey, you might want to watch this," I said.

He raised one eyebrow and didn't reply.

I thrust out my crooked right hand and introduced myself. "Hi, I'm Josh Blue."

"Yeah, kid. I know who you are."

"It's a poor recording, but you'll get the idea," I said, gesturing to the almost obsolete VHS tape. "I want to start touring, and people say you're the man I should talk to."

"How much time can you do?" he asked, but it seemed like he already knew. As I would come to discover, Mike is always one step ahead when it comes to business.

"I have a solid ten."

"That's great," he said. "Except that no one is booking anyone for ten minutes. Anywhere. Why don't we talk again when you have a solid thirty? And I can actually book you."

Instead of leaving his office feeling defeated, I was filled with a new motivation.

From there, I got on as many shows as I could, squeezing new material into the solid ten I had. Two months later, I could get away with a twenty-eight minute set. Shortly after that, I got a phone call from Mike on my first cell phone.

"Word on the street is that you are ready for me to start booking you." He took me out to lunch and explained what a manager does, and that if I worked with him, he would take ten percent of every show from then on. I agreed, and we made it official with a handshake.

"Did you ever watch that tape I gave you?" I asked.

"Ahh, no," he said, with a laugh.

After that, we spoke on a daily basis. He encouraged me to try and work clean. "I can book you on more shows for better money if you don't swear."

"The problem is when you take out all the swear words from my act, it goes back down to ten minutes," I said.

I decided on a third option. I got booked on clean gigs for good money and then fuckin' swore, anyway. I came to find that even if they wanted a clean show, if you got a standing ovation at the end, they couldn't say shit.

My hard work eventually led me to the Las Vegas Comedy Festival in October 2004. It was my first national contest, and there were a couple hundred contestants. Every evening there would be elimination rounds and, during the day, workshops on improv and stand up. It lasted four days.

Most of the workshops were taught by comedy legend Shelley Berman, an old Jewish comic who was a staple in the Borscht Belt and had been in the game, working for over seventy years. He was a delight. He had an infectious smile, a twinkle in his eye, and the biggest eyebrows that I've ever seen on a human. They stood up a good three inches off his head, and they definitely kept my attention.

In the workshop we played improv games, and he picked comics from the audience to use as volunteers. Every time he asked for a volunteer, I eagerly raised my crooked hand. It wasn't until day three that he finally picked me. I remember seeking his approval so badly. I wanted to stick out from the crowd. During the improv sketch, I did fine, but it wasn't anything to separate me from the pack.

I was one of ten comics who made it to the semi-final round. Backstage, the energy was high, and nerves were on edge. The stage director told us that Mr. Berman would be a guest judge. *This is where I'll separate myself from the pack.* And I did just that. My five-minute onstage was fire. I tried to play to the whole room, but really, I was directing all my jokes at him, taking sneak peeks to make sure he was laughing at all the right parts. To my delight, he was laughing as hard as everybody else. That performance landed me in the finals the next night.

The following morning, as all the groggy, hungover comics trickled into the workshop, Mr. Berman followed his eyebrows into the room and picked his way through the crowd to find me

"You were great last night!" he said, clapping me on the back. "I hate to admit this, but if I hadn't come to your performance, I would have talked to you condescendingly slow, like the fool in your act. I can't wait to see what you do tonight."

I was ecstatic. My improv may not have wowed him, but my stand-up had delivered. I was more interested in stand-up, anyway. I was trying to make some money.

In the final round, each contestant had ten minutes. First prize was $25,000, second place was $10,000, and third place got $2,000. This big payday had brought in serious acts from all over the country. Industry veterans with decades of experience stood around with me backstage. As expected, they all crushed, one after the other, building on each other's momentum. The able-bodied comic before me had a closing bit about an awkward interaction using the handicapped stall in a public restroom. He was encroaching on my wheelhouse, but I saw my opening.

When they introduced me, I waited a painful five to ten seconds before stumbling onstage. I theatrically wrestled the mic from the stand.

"Sorry I'm late. Some asshole was in the handicapped stall." The crowd erupted, and it was smooth sailing from there.

I was having so much fun, I ignored the light signaling that my ten minutes had come to an end. *They're having such a good time, they won't notice an extra minute or two.* But the judges did notice, and my decision to continue cost me first place.

I got second and the $10,000 prize. I'm still kicking myself at how costly that extra minute and a half was. It was a steep lesson in not running the light, but $10,000 was still the most money I had ever earned doing anything.

After the show, I went to the lobby to find Mr. Berman. He greeted me with open arms, hugged me, and said, "I knew you could do it, kid."

Later, I called Mike with the good news. He was excited and proud of me, and then he ruined it by reminding me that he gets ten percent of the winnings. "I know you're not good at math, so I'll do it for you. That's a thousand dollars."

What a buzzkill.

After the contest, Mike's confidence in my abilities became evident, as he booked me on bigger and better gigs. When I wasn't doing my own shows, I was going down to Comedy Works almost every night.

The weekend Carlos Mencia was in town, I went to see what all the hubbub was about. When I arrived at the club, there was a line around the block, waiting to see him. I pushed my way past the line, smiling to myself as people begrudgingly made way for this no-name.

I was greeted by Heather, one of my favorite servers. "Have you seen Carlos before?" she asked.

"No," I replied.

"He's a powerhouse, but he's notorious for doing painfully long shows, and all the staff hate him for that," she said. "You wanna meet him?"

"Of course I do."

We headed to the green room together.

"Hey Carlos, there's someone I want you to meet."

He stood up and made his way out into the hallway. I was surprised that he was shorter than me and wearing a soccer jersey. He had the confident energy of someone who was regularly selling out his show, and he gave me a skeptical am-I-this-guy's-Make-A-Wish-request look.

"Carlos, this is Josh Blue. He's our new up-and-coming star." Then she said in a stage whisper, "You really gotta see this kid."

"Okay, well then, let's put you on after the host. You can do as much time as you want." He shook my now sweaty hand.

And so the pacing began. I was in audience mode, ready to watch a sold-out show, and was suddenly on the bill. I was in shock at how easily Heather had gotten me in the lineup and in awe that Carlos would give a guy who looked like me an undefined time slot on his show. I decided to do seven minutes. The show was already long enough, and I feared if I made it any longer, the staff would hate me, too.

After my tight seven minutes, Carlos met me in the hallway, still laughing. "Hey kid, you can open for me anytime you want."

Six months later, Carlos came back to Comedy Works by popular demand. This was unheard of, as most comics at any club were on a year or even eighteen-month rotation. He added shows and was doing three a night, which he insisted I be on. In the green room, he told me that Comedy Central had picked up his *Mind of Mencia* show.

"You are the first person that I thought of for my show."

Yeah right.

Much to my surprise, two months later, he personally me to invite me out to L.A. to be on one of the first episodes.

His show was filmed in front of a live studio audience at the Comedy Central Studios in Los Angeles. I'd only received the script two days before and was frantically trying to learn my lines. This was going to be my first TV appearance, and I was not going to fumble.

The studio was a cold and busy place, with people adjusting all the bright lights on set and craft services refilling an unending supply of snacks. In my dressing room, I found a revised script, and the handler ushered me off to makeup and wardrobe. I was to do three sketches, playing characters such as a traffic cop and an awards presenter in a powder-blue, '70s tuxedo.

On set, the actors did the scene three times. The first was a read/walk-through, the second was a rehearsal, and the third was the recording. After a little while, in any scene where it was just Mencia and me, the director decided we could skip the rehearsal. We had such a strong rapport, and it was playing nicely on the screen.

In one sketch, we went over jobs that I was ill-qualified for. It was my first time on a green screen. I would stand there, and they could project any background behind me. One of the jobs was a chef at Benihana. They had me in a chef's hat, behind a grill filled with a mound of minced cabbage. Guests sat around and *oohed* and *aahed* as I frantically chopped with two large butcher knives, causing the cabbage to fly everywhere. Eventually, one of the knives flew out of my hand, and the camera cut to one of the guests with a prop knife sticking out of his forehead, and a thin trickle of blood running down his nose.

Watching the take with the director, he repeatedly yelled into the headset, "The part with the chopping, why is it in fast forward? Play it at regular speed." By the third time he'd said it, he was quite annoyed. Someone leaned down and said, "That is actual speed. That's just how fast his hands move."

The director took a sideways look at me that had both surprise and concern in it. With a sheepish smile and a small shrug of the shoulders, I said, "That's just the palsy quickness."

They all laughed.

The show turned out to be a hit and ran for four seasons. I was a guest in three episodes. I would have loved to do more, but I was busy with my own touring schedule and the Paralympic soccer team.

I ended up touring with Mencia as a part of his traveling

circus. He paid me $200 a show plus room and board, but I had to pay my own airfare to rendezvous with the tour bus. Many times I lost money on the trip, but what I gained was much more valuable: experience performing on huge stages.

Mencia was regularly playing to audiences of three to six thousand. What I loved the most about Mencia's shows is that I could swing the bat as hard as I could and never have to worry about him complaining that I did too well. For the next couple years, I toured with him as much as possible, interspersing as many shows with him as I could between my own gigs.

Touring on a bus was a strange experience. I felt like I never totally fit in, but it turned out that soccer was our common language. At every rest stop, gas station, and venue, we would take a break to juggle my ball. We would practice shooting by blasting the ball against the venues' loading-bay doors. Carlos loved soccer, and he was unusually agile for his chubby frame.

In the middle of touring with Carlos and traveling the world playing soccer, I was also working toward recording my first album. Part of this was battling Vocational Rehabilitation, a state government program that helped disabled folks become working members of society by giving them adaptive technology or other services that enabled them to work in their desired field.

Someone had told me that the year before, this organization had given back $2 million to the federal government, claiming they could not find any disabled people in need of their services. Which is complete bullshit.

I decided with all that money being returned, I wanted my share. But I would soon come to painfully realize why they had sent so much money back. They sent my crippled ass on a wild-goose chase, jumping through all kinds of hoops, taking tests, psychological evaluations, and physical examinations. Most of the requirements were both unfair and unrealistic for the demographic they were trying to help.

My caseworker was a blind woman nine months away from retirement, who had little to no sense of humor. It took me an hour on the bus to get to our first bullshit meeting filled with formalities and fake niceties. I presented my case of wanting to be a touring comedian. As I handed a blind woman the same VHS tape I'd given Mike, I realized how futile a venture this was going to be. She told me she would have to review what I had presented and think about ways that Vocational Rehab could help.

One week later, I was on the bus heading back to meet my caseworker. I was fantasizing about renting a full-body chicken suit to wear into my meeting. It made me laugh to think about sitting across from her, having a serious conversation about my future, while she had no idea that I was dressed up like a buffoon.

As my caseworker settled in behind her desk, I asked, "Did you review my stand-up tape?"

"No," she answered, curtly. After a painful pause, she followed with, "I've reviewed your case, and I feel like you should pursue something more realistic."

"How could you possibly know what's realistic if you haven't seen my performance?" I asked.

"It's just not a very realistic goal. I think you should pursue something more realistic," she repeated.

"Like what, flipping burgers?" I asked as my heart sank. Her blindness was not just in her eyes. The rest of the meeting went back and forth with me defending my point of view and it falling on deaf ears. The meeting ended with her telling me to go home and reboot my idea.

"We can have another meeting when you put together an idea that we can work with."

I went home fuming.

The next couple weeks, I bitched to anyone who would listen. The friend who told me about Vocational Rehab sending the money back told me that the state would provide me with a disability advocate. *Well, why didn't you tell me that in the first place?*

My disability advocate was a middle-aged man named Henry. Henry and I met for coffee, and he was as cool as a cucumber. I told him what I was trying to do and what had happened. He told me he had dealt with my caseworker before, and she was a notorious stick in the mud.

The day of my next meeting, he picked me up; no bus this time. On the drive, I joked with him, "I appreciate your help, but I think it's pretty funny that the government provides an advocate to fight themselves." He laughed. I felt confident, and he reassured me.

When we walked in, my caseworker was sitting behind the desk.

"Hello," I said, "I brought a friend."

"Hi June, it's Henry. We've worked together before. I'm Josh's advocate."

She visibly stiffened, which made me smile. Henry gave me a little wink.

"Oh, did I do something wrong?" June asked in her most innocent tone.

"Well, Josh feels like you're more of an obstacle than a guide through this process," he said.

She stiffened a little bit more.

It only took one meeting with my advocate to get June to see my potential. This started the laborious machine. They provided me with a business manager to help me write up a three-year business plan. The plan couldn't have been more spot-on in terms of a projection of the next three years, but the first year was rough.

Vocational Rehab would not be separated from its money easily. There was an endless amount of paperwork to fill out. I wasn't worried about the physical examination; I was playing on the Paralympic soccer team, which proved I was disabled. But the psychiatric evaluation almost sidelined the deal. They did tests on me that reminded me of the tests they used to pull me out of class for, from kindergarten to the twelfth grade: simple math, reading comprehension, ink blots, word association…and maybe even a little shock therapy.

The doctor gave me three elements and told me to make up a story using all of them on the spot. As usual, my story was sarcastic and dry, and it was apparent that he didn't get my brand of humor. Later, June gleefully told me his evaluation was that stand-up wouldn't be a realistic job for me because my storytelling ability was poor, and no one would be able to follow what I was saying.

"Well, yeah, there's a big difference between telling a couple hundred people a joke and telling someone who is already not on my side a story. And besides, he's not my target audience," I explained. "Do we need Henry to come back here?"

June granted me the funding.

I ended up receiving just under $20,000 in equipment and funding. I purchased a new computer with voice recognition, a printer and scanner, and a brand-new flip phone. A large portion of the money went toward producing my first album, *Good Josh, Bad Arm*, which I recorded at Comedy Works in Denver.

Now I had something to sell after the shows, and I learned that's where comics make most of their money. It was a game-changer. I was selling CDs for ten bucks after the show, a CD that I paid nothing to have printed. If I sold five CDs, that would be an extra $50. That money was the oil that kept the touring machine going. I could spend that money for food on the road and then afford to buy plane tickets to get to the next gig.

However, many gig headliners will not let their opening act sell after the show, and Mencia was no different. This helped form one of my philosophies on the road: always let your opener sell their stuff. Knowing how big the pay gap between opener and headliner is, and knowing what it was like to be in that position, I don't want to forget where I came from.

()()()

Mike entered me in the NACA showcase. NACA is the National Association of Campus Activities. Every year they have several regional events and one big national showcase where desperate artists from musicians to magicians to ventriloquists pay to show off their talent in hopes of getting booked at high-paying college gigs. I ended up getting seventh alternate for the national showcase in Boston. That meant six people would have to drop out—or in the case of magicians, I hoped, die—in order for me to get a chance at the big stage.

Sure enough, one by one acts started to drop out. I got down to second alternate. Mike and I decided I should go in case the last two didn't make it, and good thing I did. I ended up landing a fifteen-minute, main-stage showcase in front of over two hundred

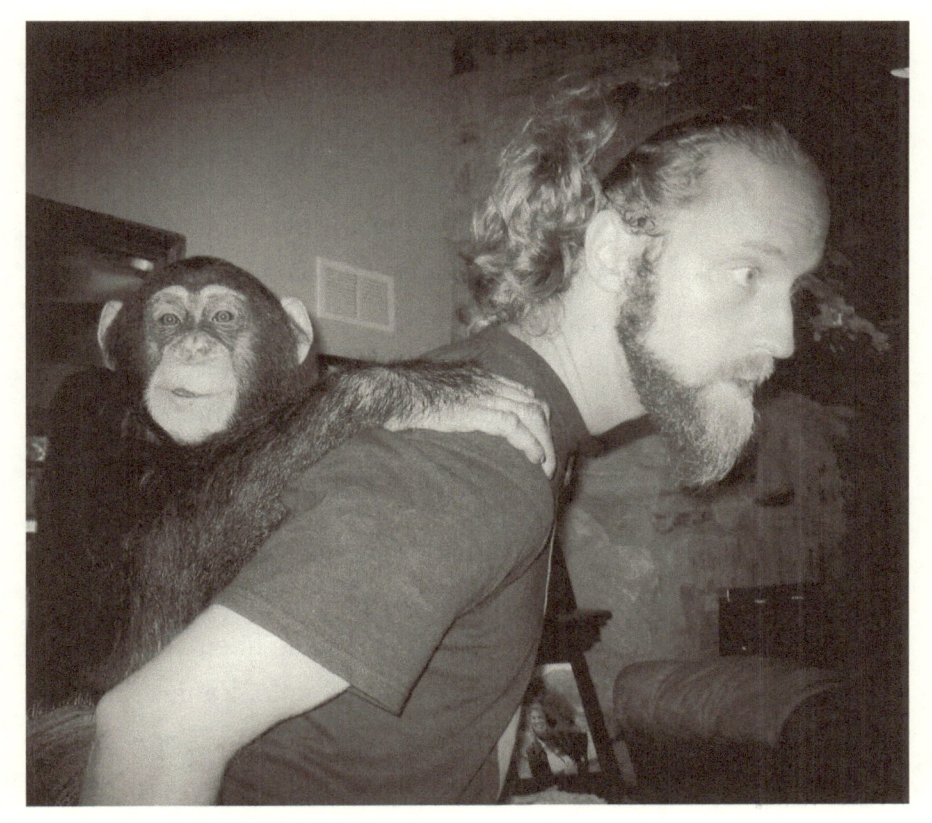

I always make time for my fans.

schools. I didn't squander the opportunity. My brand of humor was perfect for that audience. I was in my mid-twenties, but I was something they hadn't seen before. Also, I was ideal for filling the diversity quota of many colleges.

For a lot of it, Mike was stressing, "Don't swear, be clean, be good." I wasn't worried. For me, it goes back to playing by the rules until you don't have to. Be a clean act, and then, when you get there, give the students what they want.

From that one showcase, I ended up booking fifty well-paid but difficult gigs. Difficult because I'd come to find that, for a place of higher learning, there were a lot of dumb motherfuckers there. Within the next year and a half, I wasn't able to honor all the gigs I'd gotten at NACA because a much larger opportunity was coming my way.

Shortly after NACA, I was standing in line in Chicago to try out for the reality TV show *Last Comic Standing*, which is kind of like *The Real World* but for comics. In the show, a cast of comedians live together and complete challenges as well as perform stand-up to become the proverbial last comic standing. It was three o'clock in the morning and minus 15 degrees. There were hundreds of comics in line, freezing their jokes off, waiting to audition. Despite the constant reminder of the time and temperature from the bank clock across the street, spirits were high and I could hear laughter up and down the line.

At 7 a.m., the first hopefuls were let into Zanies Comedy Club. Daylight broke over the sluggish line. At 10, a representative from the TV show came and cut the line off two people behind me, saying these were all the comics they would have time for. A groan went down the line.

When I made it into the club, my feet were blocks of ice. They had us warm up by doing a mountain of paperwork. The handlers briefed us on the rules of engagement and shrugged off our many nervous questions. Each comic was given two minutes to try to dazzle the two judges and a cameraman. The handlers emphasized that the judges were also the people in charge of booking *The Tonight Show*, to add a little extra pressure—knowing if you messed up, your chances for *The Tonight Show* were gone as well.

The comics were treated like herd animals. When paperwork was done, we were prodded into the line leading to the butcher block. Each step of the way brought more questions from us about the process, but we were deliberately kept in the dark. I just wanted a glimpse of the stage to know what I was walking into.

The doors opened, and we were ushered into the empty showroom, flooded with overly bright lights. I wished the comic in front of me luck as he took the plunge. When he was up there, I strained my ears to hear the laughter that never came. His two minutes went by painfully, for both of us. The nervous knot in my stomach was about to burst.

As I pulled the mic from the stand, I told them my name and where I was from. The two judges, bored at this point in the day, told me to proceed.

I started right in, "You know, people ask me if I get nervous coming up onstage, I say, 'Heck no, I got this many people staring at me all day.'"

The judge on the left feigned a smile, while the judge on the right seemed to be checking emails. I quickly realized that a joke is a lot funnier when there are more than two people in the audience.

Rattled, I stumbled into the next joke. "When I was a kid, my mom told me if I went on a roller coaster, my head would snap off—"

They stopped me there.

"Thank you, we've seen enough," said Email judge.

"Can I at least get to the punchline?" I asked.

"Thanks, we're good," said the other judge. I fumbled the microphone back into the stand and tried to hold my head high as a handler escorted me past the judges and toward the exit. As I wobbled past, I looked at them sternly and said, "Well, this is a shitty Make-A-Wish."

They both laughed.

LAST COMIC STANDING: TRY, TRY AGAIN

In hindsight, I'm glad they didn't pick me. I wasn't ready. I will admit I left with a chip on my shoulder. *Well, fuck you, I'll show you how good I am.* Then I went out and did a lot of college shows and really paid my dues, doing an hour at a different school a few nights a week.

College audiences were by no means a slam dunk. The shows were put on by the campus, and admission was free, so half the crowd might be bored students who just wandered in and could wander right back out. The majority were also painfully sober, so there was no booze greasing the gears. The schools often had no experience putting on a comedy show, and it would be held in a terrible location, such as an active cafeteria or echoing gymnasium. Once I had to perform from the center of a soccer pitch while the audience sat seventy-five yards away in the bleachers, straining into the sun to see me. I would often call Mike before a show in a panic, and he would talk me off the ledge. He would remind me that it's all about collecting a paycheck.

"Yeah, but you aren't the one out here collecting it," I'd retort.

"You're good at what you do, and you'll be fine."

All in all, these colleges were the perfect place to refine my headlining set. I felt like I had come full circle from my first time performing at the housing community center at Evergreen. Now I could perform anywhere, from a church to a barn to an airplane hangar.

The next year I really didn't want to go back to audition for *Last Comic Standing* because 1) I didn't think they were looking for real talent, and 2) I didn't want to get rejected again. I told people, "It's just a dumb reality show." But Mike insisted I try again.

Mike procured an audition for me at Caroline's in New York City, and I didn't have to wait in line in the freezing cold this time. It was a scheduled audition, with the same two judges. Caroline's is a legendary club in Manhattan, and I had never been there. The walls were covered with framed headshots from the biggest names in comedy history. I was visibly nervous, but they let me get through my entire two minutes.

The first judge asked the other, "Did you like him?"

"Yeah, he has a unique perspective," Email judge answered and then turned to me, "we'll see you tonight."

The night performance was a live, sold-out show. Even if the judges didn't like the performer, if the audience laughed, the comics couldn't be denied. This time I had five minutes instead of two, which makes a world of difference. I was there to get the chip off my shoulder. Between the audition in Chicago and this one, I had done over two hundred shows across the country, most of which I'd headlined, but a lot of which I'd opened for Mencia in front of giant audiences. I had diversified and grown as a comic. My joke writing was stronger, and my confidence onstage had developed by leaps and bounds.

My competition this time was professional touring comics, not a bunch of half-frozen amateurs that stood in line all day. When my set was done, I took a little bow and waited with the rest of the comics to hear our fate. When it came time, all fifteen of us went back onstage and stood in a tight, anxious knot. I knew I had done well, but there were still things that could go wrong. *What if the judges have it out for me? What if I have gone over my time? What if my fly was down?*

They told us five comics would advance from New York. They picked me fifth. The intentional suspense almost killed me. They handed me what they called The Golden Ticket in a red envelope. The crowd went wild, and I jumped offstage. If I could do a cartwheel, I would have. That envelope was my ticket to the Los Angeles auditions, which would determine whether I was a cast member or not. In the lobby, I eagerly ripped it open. Empty. I went from ecstatic to panic before I realized that just like waiting in line in Chicago—it was all for the cameras.

A few weeks later, I landed at LAX and was met by a guy with a clipboard. He was there to pick up the forty comedian contestants from all over the nation. He had very little information about or interest in all of my questions.

"How long will my set be? What comedian do I have to share a room with? Will there be craft services?"

He told me to get in the van. "You'll be fully informed when you get to the hotel."

At the hotel, there was a registration table and more paperwork. After that, they encouraged the comics to eat lunch together. It was extremely annoying with everyone trying to one-up each other, and the cameras weren't even rolling yet. There was one comic who was high on his horse about having a clean act. Between spoonfuls of lunch, he told us how he prided himself on not having to use any swear words to get his point across. I finally responded, "What the fuck are you talkin' about?" He was the only one to not laugh.

Roz laughed the loudest. She was one of the comics who had advanced with me from New York. When I was there, I gravitated toward her, maybe because she weighed three hundred pounds, and she had an even bigger personality. She was funny onstage and off. I remember her opening joke was, "I ain't got jokes, I got prohhhblemsss." She reminded me of Miss Daniels from back in school. They were both strong Black women, and their presence commanded respect.

I tried to meet all of my competition. There were so many personalities and comics that went on to be big names, like Doug Benson, Tig, and Nikki Glaser, the youngest person ever to advance. Everyone seemed more than a little nervous. Nobody knew what was going on, but at least we were all lost together.

Another comic who advanced from New York was Joey Gay. He had a thick New York accent and a glowing energy behind it. That night, we walked to our first event together. On the way, we talked about where we were from. We made each other laugh. *Wow, this guy's really sweet.* As we got to the door where all the lights and cameras were, Joey turned to me and said, "It was a pleasure talking to you. Now you'll have to excuse me. I'm going to go and be a loud-mouthed asshole."

There wasn't much direction to the event. They told us a few logistical things, and that they just wanted to catch us all mingling. They needed a bunch of B-roll. In the hour and a half they had us there, I drank as many free beers as I could and tried to avoid the loud-mouthed asshole. But the cameras loved him, and he was getting most of their attention. *Do I need to do that?* I decided to stay in my corner and fling snide remarks. There were quite a few other bright personalities that shined in that setting, and I realized there were two layers of performance I'd have to give: the stand-up onstage and shining the brightest among the comics offstage.

Later that night, after the cameras were off and the hotel

stopped serving beer, a group of us risked being kicked off the show by sneaking across the street to the liquor store. We were filming the next day, and I find it best to perform on a hangover. We had all made it this far, but after tomorrow's show, more than half of us would be eliminated.

Our day was filled with more paperwork. In mid-afternoon, they filmed us getting onto school buses and heading off to the Alex Theater.

When we arrived, I was surprised to see there was already a line around the block. The show wasn't for four hours. I discovered that making reality television is a lot of hurry up and wait. Unlike a regular stand-up show where all you need is a microphone and an audience, a simple reality TV show has a lot of moving parts.

We waited for our chance to advance in big canvas tents set up in the parking lot. There were going to be two shows that night, with two different audiences and three celebrity judges: Gary Marshall, Kathy Griffin, and Tim Meadows. Twenty of us would be on each show. Post editing, each show would be presented to the public as a different episode by host and comic Anthony Clark.

I found out I was to do my five minutes somewhere in the middle of the second show, giving me plenty of time to pace and panic. I picked at the buffet and ate what my stomach would allow—not much. There were big screen TVs in the tents for us to watch our competition. It made me more nervous. I reflected on how weird it was that comedy was a competition, because humor is subjective. But when you can get a room full of strangers to laugh at the same thing, that's where the beauty lies. No matter what your background is, a laugh is a laugh.

As nervous as I was offstage, the second I stepped into the

lights, the feeling turned into raw energy, and I was free to do what I love: make people laugh. Directly in front of me was a giant, flat-screen TV that had a digital timer and counted down my five minutes. If I went over my time, they cut the microphone. This happened to Chris Porter, a really funny comic who went on shortly before me. When he came offstage, he was visibly shaken, thinking he had ruined his chance. I had learned my lesson in Vegas and was not going to make the same mistake. The time flew by with electric laughter that made me want to push past my time, but I said goodnight in the nick of time. The crowd roared, and the judges asked me to stay onstage.

Kathy Griffin asked me why I wanted to do stand-up. Without missing a beat, I said, "I didn't really have a choice. What am I gonna do? Be a traffic cop?" This was already on the tip of my brain from having just done the sketch with Mencia. The crowd lost their minds and gave me a full standing ovation, which no one had received yet. I bounded offstage to seek the praise of my competition. In my heart, I knew I was advancing, but it was a reality TV show, and they could edit it however they wanted.

At the end of the night, it was Roz, Chris Porter, Joey Gay, Michele Balan, and me. As the audience favorite, I was also $1,000 richer. From the other show, Gabriel Iglesias, Stella Stolper, Ty Barnett, Bill Dwyer, and April Macie were selected. In a special twist, Rebecca Corry and Kristin Key were also chosen, because the judges couldn't decide.

All the finalists had a couple weeks to go home, pack, and prepare before boarding the *Queen Mary*—a notoriously haunted cruise ship from the '30s.

For the first time, maybe ever, I did go home and prepare.

But first, a detour to Mexico. I happened to have a family trip already planned to visit my sister Emily on Isla Mujeres. I sat on the beach and reflected on how this was probably the last time I would be able to go anywhere without being recognized. I learned by watching successful comics over the last few years how people change around success. When you're a funny comic but a no-name, people come and tell you that you're funny, but when you're a funny comic and successful, people no longer tell you that you're funny, they just tell you who you are. Shortly after that, a tourist on the beach told me who I was. "Hey, you're Josh Blue!"

"Bitch, I know!"

When I got back stateside, I hit the ground running. I met with a group of comics to stock me up on new jokes. Part of the deal on *Last Comic Standing* was no outside contact once the show started. This included phones of any kind. I wasn't sure how much material I would burn through, and I wanted to have enough jokes where I would never have to repeat myself. Some of the jokes I did on *Last Comic Standing* I had never done before and never did again.

John Heffron, the winner of Season 2, happened to be playing Comedy Works the week before I moved into the *Queen Mary*. Mike set up a meeting with him. We sat around a conference table and grilled him about everything he wished he'd known before he won. John was gracious and helpful. I left the meeting with more confidence and eager to get this thing rolling.

()()()

A helicopter with a camera crew followed us on our short bus to the *Queen Mary*. I thought it was pretty funny that our transport was a short bus. Advantage: me. When we pulled up to the *Queen Mary*, we were all taken aback by how old the ship looked—a creepy, kitschy hotel, cemented to the pier.

From this point on, we were being filmed 24/7. Cameras were hidden all through the ship, and camera people followed us to capture our every waking and sleeping moments. They followed us everywhere but the bathroom.

My roommate was Gabriel Iglesias, who I felt was my biggest opponent, literally and figuratively. Gabriel weighed over 300 pounds and was a pretty well-established stand-up on the scene, known for his characters and impressions. He carried me over the threshold like newlyweds, and we were all smiles as the camera ate us up. Then he unceremoniously threw me on the bed—the honeymoon was over.

We were all sizing each other up, and the consensus was that none of us liked Stella Stolper. She was arrogant and mean-spirited, ultimately marking herself a target for elimination. In sticking with the making of good television, the producers had her room with Roz, and Roz hated her guts. They were at each other from the get-go. They were both excessively loud, and by the end of day one, I thought they were going to come to blows, which would have been bad because Stella was seven months pregnant.

The first night on the ship, we had a formal dinner. We all dressed up in our finest; I wore my blue pinstripe suit, which I had bought two days before boarding the ship. It was my first suit that wasn't from Goodwill.

At the table, Rebecca Corry made a toast, "No matter what happens, we all made it this far and congratulations."

We hoisted our glasses.

Stella followed with, "No matter what happens, I'm not

scared of any of you bitches."

Nobody cheered.

Chris Porter followed with a final toast, "Here's to Stella being a bitch."

We all raised our glasses high. "Hear, hear!"

Our first event was the heckler challenge. They paired us up, and we each had six minutes to do stand-up while the other person sat in the audience and rained down insults. Then the roles were reversed. My opponent was Chris Porter, who I had been gravitating toward. Chris is very tall and looks like Willy Wonka. We are birthday buddies, born on the exact same day of the same year, on opposite sides of the planet. We both have a biting sense of humor and love to smoke weed, which was strictly prohibited on the show. We commiserated about this.

He was a worthy opponent and ultimately won the entire heckler challenge, gaining immunity in the head-to-head that night: two comics had six-minute sets to prove they were worthy of staying on the ship, and the audience would decide which one of them would go home.

The comics that were to perform were chosen by us, the contestants. One by one, we went into a room with a camera, sat down in a chair, and said, "I know I'm funnier than ____." I knew I was funnier than Stella, and many of the others felt they were, too. In the end, it was a tie between Stella and Michele Balan. Because it was a tie, Michele and Stella got to pick a third person. They picked April Macie. A wave of relief crashed over the rest of us: We would not have to perform that night. Now all we had to do was eat catered food, drink free booze, and watch and hope that Stella would get eliminated.

They loaded us up on the short bus and took us back to the Alex Theater. For maximum drama, the three performers had to bring their packed bags with them. Whoever was eliminated would leave immediately, never to be seen again. The three women on the chopping block looked gaunt and worried, while the rest of us were enjoying a night off and trying not to think of what challenges the next day would bring. Kristin Key and I sat together and drank beer from a giant cooler. By the end of the night, April and Stella were eliminated, and Kristin and I were drunk.

Later, on the boat, Michele was still in shock that she had advanced. "I thought they'd eliminate the old person first," she said in her raspy New York accent.

Frankly, we were all stunned that she had beaten April Macie. I passed out and was unpleasantly surprised to be woken up a few hours later at 3 a.m. with a camera in my face. We had forty minutes to prepare and be on the bus, ready for our next challenge. I was definitely still half-drunk. On the bus, I pulled my headband over my eyes and tried to sleep it off in rush hour traffic, which occurs even before dawn in L.A.

An hour and a half later, we showed up at Adam Corolla's morning radio show. In the waiting room, we were given manila folders. Inside, we each found a different, fake magazine. The challenge was to make up a minute of material based on the phony magazine, and we had to do it live on Adam's show. It was brutal. My magazine was *Weapons of Death,* and my first reaction, "Aren't all weapons for death?"

Chris Porter's publication was in Spanish.

I spent my minute with Adam, trying to chat about other things. I said, "Hey Adam, this really sucks."

He replied, "Yeah, how do you think me and my listeners feel?"

Kristin Key did the best by far, considering her magazine was *Modern Knitting*. She only did thirty-eight seconds of the requisite minute, so Adam robbed her and gave the win to Rebecca Corry, which in turn gave her immunity for that night's head-to-head. She spent the rest of the day reminding everyone how she was untouchable.

That day we had a lot of time to kill before the head-to-head, so Kristin and I invented a game called crotchball. The rules were simple. We stood facing each other, twelve feet apart. I had a soccer ball, and she had a crotch; she had her hands clasped behind her back and feet shoulder-width apart; I took free kicks and tried to hit her in the hoo-ha. We played for hours. Coach Hoffman would be happy to know I got my practice in. The best part was that this was the entire game—the roles were never reversed.

For ambiance in the bowels of the ship, they had candlelight and a fog machine that randomly let out loud bursts of steam. It set off my palsy reflex every time, to the delight of everyone but me. I went with it, over-exaggerating and pretending I was in a bad episode of *Scooby-Doo*, screaming "Zoinks!" with every blast. They got me three times on the walk down the bridge to the confessional.

Once in the room, I put on my secret disguise: some glasses I had taped in the middle and knocked the lenses out of. I slacked my jaw and bucked my teeth as I peered owlishly into the camera and said in a scared moron's voice, "I think I'm funnier than

Gabriel." Then I looked around the room and said, almost to myself, "Oh Lord, what have I done?" and ran out.

My strategy was to pick Gabriel, because I knew no one else would. He was clearly one of the biggest threats in the competition and also the *biggest* threat in the competition. My strategy had the unintended bonus of letting the other contestants know that if I wasn't scared of him, I wasn't scared of any of them.

That night I sat next to Kristin in the creepy boiler room with the other comics, waiting to say who we were funnier than. She was still sore, not (just) from the game of crotchball, but from losing immunity. At this point in the competition, we were feeling a bit more comfortable—or maybe we all gave a little less of a shit.

We all had a laugh watching everyone say who they were funnier than. People were more playful despite the pressure of the looming head-to-head. Everyone put on their own mini-performance in the confessional, trying to make an awkward situation as funny as possible. Bill Dwyer mentioned something about usable fire exits and then did a pratfall. Gabriel put everyone's name in a hat and picked a random. He did this every time, showing us that he wasn't afraid. Everyone laughed at my silly glasses. When I said I was funnier than Gabriel, everyone but him sucked in a sharp breath. Gabriel remained casual and calm. He radiated the energy of someone who expected to win it all. It ended up being a four-way tie between Chris Porter, Joey Gay, Bill Dwyer, and Michele Balan, which the producers were not planning for. By the end of the night, Bill Dwyer and Joey Gay went home, and Kristin and I were drunk again.

We had all been happy to see Stella go, but as more comics were being voted off, I was sad to see them leave. Although, it was also a great relief it wasn't me.

The next day, we were all visibly exhausted as they explained our next challenge. We were to roast one of our own. We all voted on the roastee. Gabriel won, or lost, depending on how you look at it. He was a big target.

That night, at the Friar's Club in Beverly Hills, the eight remaining comics sat on the dais as the Roastmaster Jim Norton introduced the celebrity judges. The first judge was the wonderful Phyllis Diller, who looked like a reanimated corpse. I knew she was a legendary comedian from the dark ages, but I recognized her more from her numerous cameos on *Scooby-Doo*. Next was the grating Gilbert Gottfried, best known perhaps as the parrot from *Aladdin* or the Aflac Duck. An annoying bird either way. The third judge was Alonzo Bodden, who had won Season 3 of *Last Comic Standing* and had somehow conned his way next to Diller and Gottfried.

I went first and asked Gabriel how much money he got for his tusks. I followed it up with, "They say you are what you eat. That poor Vietnamese family."

In a roast the usual rules of decorum go out the window, and you generally pick on the easiest and most obvious traits of the roastee, and with Gabriel it was his weight. I closed my bit by mentioning that Gabriel and I were roommates and then said, "You know you're fat when you start snoring *before* you're asleep!" This was my first roast ever, and I walked back to my seat, feeling like I had really held my own.

Every one of us laid it on thick with the fat jokes, and Gabriel (jelly) rolled with the punches, laughing along. In true roast fashion, we went after each other as well. Ty said I would be a terrible sniper. Kristin referred to Michele as an old catcher's mitt.

At the end, Gabriel got to fire back at all of us, and he gave as good as he got. He had absorbed a heaping amount of insults but, like any fat kid, was ready to fire back.

Finally, we heard from the judges. Gilbert Gottfried told me, "Your jokes are so bad, you should go blind, too." I laughed so hard I had to put my head on the table. No wonder they fired that asshole from being the Aflac Duck.

In the end, Chris Porter won the roast, which really meant nothing, because there was no more immunity. The next day was the final head-to-head. Three comics would compete, and one would stay for the finals. Now, gentle reader, if this all sounds confusing to you, believe me, it was even more confusing to us. In classic reality-show fashion, the rules and format seemed to change on the fly.

The next morning, we had some downtime to mentally prepare. Kristin and I were playing a lively round of crotchball, when suddenly there was some commotion near Gabriel. I walked over and saw the big guy trying to hide an object. One of the cameramen was up in his business, badgering him.

"Heeey, whatcha got there? Is that a cell phone?"

It turned out Gabriel had been caught on camera texting, which was expressly forbidden. By the look on his face, he knew he was busted. It was like seeing a walrus caught with his flipper in the oyster jar.

The producers scrambled; this threw a wrench in their production. Gabriel was clearly in the running to be a finalist, and they did not want to lose him. But the rules were clear: no outside contact with anyone, to ensure you weren't receiving any outside help.

Later, they discovered he had also broken curfew and snuck

out of our room at three in the morning. As his roommate, I was surprised to hear any of this. But I also kind of wondered why he had a phone charger in the bathroom.

That night in the boiler room, Gabriel did not show up. In dramatic form, Anthony Clark explained to the comedians and the cameras that Gabriel Iglesias had been kicked off the boat for cheating, which was greeted by a mixed response. We were sad that our friend was gone, but relieved that there was one less powerhouse to contend with. They expected us to go on our merry way, eliminating more friends.

I said I was funnier than Ty, and Chris Porter said he was funnier than me. In the end, it was Ty, Kristin, and Rebecca off to the final head-to-head-to-head. This meant that Chris, Roz, Michele, and I advanced to the Final Five and would be joined by the winner of that night's show. Ty clearly outperformed the other two, but I was super sad to see my drinking and crotchball partner leave. I would have to find a new hobby. None of the remaining contestants were going to let me boot soccer balls at their crotch.

FINALS

Making the finals meant we no longer had to stay on the *Queen Mary*. We were free to do as we pleased. From now on, we would only compete doing stand-up sets for the next four episodes, and America would be voting on who was eliminated.

The next weekend, I had six sold-out shows at The Laff Stop in Houston, at the end of which I received the biggest check thus far in my career. Since I never had to do stand-up defending myself in the head-to-heads on the *Queen Mary*, I was eager to tune up my act and happy that I had so much unused material in the bank.

Every airport, liquor store, and other liquor store I went to, people stopped me by name and wished me good luck in the finals, which would be back in L.A. the following week at the Pasadena Civic Auditorium.

The opening of the show had a helicopter circling high over Los Angeles. It cut to Chris, Ty, Roz, and Michele inside the helicopter, clutching each other in terror. Then it cut to me, at the controls, looking wilder than usual in a pair of dark, Joe Biden aviator sunglasses.

Anthony Clark reintroduced us and laid down the rules. Each comic would have five minutes of straight stand-up, and one comic would go home. Now it was time for America to decide who would be the last comic standing. The audience could vote by calling 1-877-FUNNY and entering the number associated with the comic they liked.

Anthony announced that Roz would go first. A tough spot. Her set was not well-received, and she used several jokes she'd done in a previous episode. Ty went second and had a solid set.

People held signs up in the audience like, "Ty's my guy!" Each comic had several signs, but none of them were real. They were made up by some poor PA on set and placed in the hands of the audience members, whether they liked the comic or not. Television, baby!

Anthony Clark got the energy up and introduced me. "Coming to the stage, please welcome Paula Abdul's neurosurgeon and my lover, Josh Blue!"

That made me laugh as I took the stage. All my nervousness disappeared when I was met by a wall of love; everyone stood up and clapped. I had received standing ovations after my set, but this was the first time I was greeted by one. Their energy was so strong, I couldn't help but beam, and I felt a surge of adrenaline. There were a lot of fake elements to the show, but the crowd's response was real. In that moment, I realized these people had been supporting me all season, and now here they were in the flesh. Even though I had barely done actual stand-up on the show, they had bonded with my personality and crotchball skills.

When the audience settled enough for me to speak, my five minutes had been whittled down to four. I said something about how exciting it was to be there, and then feigned embarrassment as I said, "I'm so sorry everyone," and fumbled through the pocket of my suit for something.

When I finally extricated my cell phone and painfully flipped it open, I brought it to my ear and yelled, "Stop calling me, Gabriel!"

The crowd went absolutely insane, and I rode the wave on down to the end of my set for another standing ovation. Coming offstage, I could not have felt better.

The next week went by like a hurricane: plane rides, photo shoots, and autographs. Before I knew it, I was back in the Pasadena Civic Auditorium, and we were saying goodbye to Roz. In dramatic form, they brought us all out onstage and dragged out the agony, announcing who would stay to perform that night until it was whittled down to Roz and Michele. When they announced Roz was going home, Michele staggered back in shock as Roz tried to be a good sport.

Backstage we all hugged Roz for a long time as Gary Gulman, a comic from Season 2, warmed up the audience. Michele went first. Most of her set was about being shocked she was still on the show, and saying thank you to the voters. I was second, and I strutted out onstage in my Paralympic soccer jersey with my name on the back. Again, I was met by a roaring crowd already on their feet.

My whole set was about my adventures traveling with the team. The bit that pushed it over the top was when I was injured during the last game, and my coach had the nerve to put me on the "disabled" list. This was my beautiful game: my timing was impeccable, and I didn't feel rushed in my five minutes. As confident as I felt in my set, I knew I had to wait an agonizing week to find out if I had advanced.

The following week was more of the same, and bouncing city to city like a human ping-pong ball was my new normal. The vibe traveling that week made me confident I would advance, and I was right; we finally got rid of Michele. She hung on like a New York cockroach, but her number was up. It was sad to say goodbye to the old catcher's mitt, but it also meant I was one step closer to winning it all.

I saw Kristin Key in the audience before the show, and as we made eye contact, I pantomimed kicking a ball at her. Chris, Ty, and I collectively snuck out of our dressing rooms to smoke weed in the parking lot; a tradition we'd been doing since we made the finals. We all had solid sets, except Chris repeated several jokes from earlier in the season, which I had learned was certain death in this competition.

The next week, in dramatic form, they sent my birthday buddy Chris home, but not before dragging it out by having three comics perform. It turns out comedians Theo Von and Josh Wolf were in a competition I didn't know existed, *Last Comic Downloaded,* the online version of *Last Comic Standing,* using comics who had been eliminated earlier in the season in the audition phase. Anthony Clark wrapped up, "Vote online now for Theo Von or Josh Wolf, and we'll find out which of them is the winner, on our season finale!"

I didn't give a shit about their competition. I just wanted to know if I would be at the season finale. The anticipation had my guts in a grinder and my armpits slick as I waited in the wings with Ty and Chris. My anxiety was at its peak.

"Soon we'll find out which one of our finalists will go home tonight. But first, one of the Latin Kings of Comedy, Paul Rodriguez!"

"Arrg," I said, as our buzz was wearing off. I joked with the guys, "Hey, you think this means we have time to smoke some more weed?"

After Paul finished, Anthony invited the three of us onstage.

"Now is the moment we've all been waiting for! We'll find out which two of these comics are going to the finals and which one will go home. Right after this commercial break!"

Right before they switched it to a commercial, you can see me bent at the waist, hands on knees, visibly frustrated. During the break, I saw my parents in the audience.

"We should've smoked that bowl," I said to the guys. You could see a slight ring forming in my armpits. When we came back from break, we were all fidgety and had trouble keeping our marks onstage.

Anthony Clark theatrically walked back and forth, looking us up and down, eventually stopping at Chris and telling him he was the one heading home. We all hugged and shook hands. Chris had become my best friend on the show, and what he had done thus far would catapult his career beyond anything he had seen.

Now that I had been through that trauma, Ty and I had five minutes to prepare to perform again, as Anthony took us into another commercial break.

At this point, I was using my material sparingly; I had saved the best for last. I had plenty of jokes, but I didn't want to use them because I was about to go on the tour of my life, and I didn't want the audience to hear the same shit again.

The crowd was with me, as always. They had an energy that only finals could bring out, but I was off; my timing was missing its mark, and the comfortable air I had the previous two weeks was gone. I pandered my way through the first few minutes, and throughout the set I used my crooked arm like a prop, waving it around in place of jokes. But they laughed anyway, more out of obligation than from the heart. I don't know why I was off. Perhaps it was seeing my birthday buddy get eliminated, or I was just finally feeling the pressure of a reality TV competition. The stakes had never been higher than this performance.

I paced the stage, nervous, watching my five minutes click away. If I went over, they would cut the mic, but this time I wasn't worried about running the light. I was worried about my planned set even hitting five minutes.

I stopped and stood alone on the huge stage. My set hadn't been going to plan. I had been coasting on the show, and this was the first time I felt challenged all season. If I was going to get back on track, it was now or never. In that moment, I harnessed all my experience in comedy—from goofing around at Evergreen to headlining clubs and colleges coast to coast—and steadied myself. I didn't make it this far to go out on a sub-par performance. I went into the joke I'd been saving for this moment.

"You know, it's great having a disability. I can get away with pretty much anything I want. I can talk trash to anybody. Cuz what are you gonna do? Beat me up? That's not something you can go home and brag about. 'Hey Larry, come here! Last night I went to a comedy show, and I kicked the crap out of a cripple!' My luck, I would find someone who *would* beat me up. And hit me in the right spot…and fix me! There goes my gig! Can you imagine if I didn't have cerebral palsy?" I wanted to say, then I'd have to tell dick jokes like the rest of these fuckers, but due to television regulations, I had to improvise. "Then I'd have to tell genital jokes like the rest of these guys!" I gestured toward the back of the stage. The crowd was eating it up as I came into the home stretch.

The clock was now counting down the final seconds. I finished with, "You don't want to mess with me though because I have this thing I like to call the Palsy Punch. First of all," I wildly swung my right arm forward, "you don't know where it's coming from. Second of all, neither do I!"

The crowd roared with the authentic laughter that I had been missing all set and finally tapped into. It was a perfectly placed one-timer goal in overtime.

"Thank you all, I love you all so much!" I said, as the final seconds ticked away, and Anthony Clark came back out. I meant what I said. I had felt the love of America, the entire country, over the course of the season, from gas stations in the middle of nowhere, to airports, to just random people on the street. It was crazy to feel so much support from a country. In that set, I had faith I would find that connection with America again, and I did.

Instead of waiting a whole painful week this time, the show would conclude in two days, which was still agony. Ty's set was strong; he had also saved his best stuff for last. At no point in the competition did I ever feel like these were my enemies, except for Stella. This was a friendly competition with very high stakes. Even bigger than the Paralympics. I've been exhausted at the end of soccer matches, but this was different. We had been competing for months, and tonight we would finally find out who would go home with the medal and the money. There was $35,000 on the line.

Just like the Paralympics, my parents had come to support me, and I desperately wanted to provide them with a better outcome than I did in Greece. I didn't get to see them outside of the venue during the grand finale because they had Ty and me sequestered in our hotel. We spent the day together, bouncing between our hotel rooms smoking weed to ensure we would both get charged the smoke-cleaning fee. We listened to music, reminisced about our journey, and wished the other luck.

The final episode was live, and the energy was more intense than the previous final episodes, which I didn't think was possible.

Anthony Clark was noticeably hungover and sounded like he was ready to be done with this shit as he introduced Ty and me. We entered down the aisles of the theater. The crowd was on its feet, clapping. All the former contestants from the show were there in the audience, even Stella. We slapped high fives with the fans on our way up onto the stage. As we stood beside Anthony Clark, Ty and I realized we were wearing almost the exact same outfit, something only two stoner buddies could do.

Anthony Clark introduced some never-before-seen footage from when all the contestants were quarantined aboard the *Queen Mary*. The producers set up a seance in the abandoned pool in the bowels of the boat. They had us crawl down into the dry pool and sit around a candlelit table while a shitty magician tried to scare us. We all rolled our eyes watching him bomb magician-style, and Roz just glared daggers at him. If you know anything, you know that comics despise magicians.

He told us that fifty-two souls had died on the ship. The reel cut to me in an interview saying, "What a [shitty] cruise line." They bleeped the word shitty, but I still got my point across. He whispered that a little girl had drowned in the pool that we were now in as he produced a small jar containing her ashes. More eye-rolling. It cut away to Chris saying, "Who just gives some random pedophile their daughter's ashes?"

Seeing that his audience was not loving his performance, the magician tried to do some tricks with a rope. The edit cut to me, fumbling with a big rope that I'd found on the boat. "If you move your hands around like this, then you can tie a knot!"

It cut back to the live episode with Ty and me waiting onstage and to the audience laughing.

"In a minute we'll hear these two comics' last performance,

and at the end we'll find out who is the LAST...COMIC...STANDING!"

After a commercial break, Anthony Clark introduced Dat Phan, the Season 1 winner. Dat did his five minutes, and then Anthony introduced John Heffron. He did ten minutes, and he killed it. After his set, they cut backstage to Ty and me, sitting nervously next to each other, our eyes bloodshot from all the weed we'd smoked that day.

Then more stand up from Alonzo Bodden. He had been on two seasons of the show. In his set, he talked about how it was better to be number one, or number three, but coming in second was the worst. "When you get third place, they do a montage of highlights of your time on the show. But if you get second place, you stand here," he planted himself at the back of the stage, "as everyone celebrates the winner."

Peter Engel, one of the producers of this show and the award-winning *Saved by the Bell,* gave a thank you speech, and then introduced the other producer and creator of the show, as well as the original host Jay Mohr. Jay took the stage to do a five-minute set with all the poise and presence that Anthony Clark did not have. His outfit was as sharp as his stand-up.

During Jay's set, I'd come up with an idea and was frantically looking for a rope. It was also to distract me from my nerves. I knew the votes were already in, and there was nothing I could do to change the outcome, but it's that damn waiting.

Ty and I shook hands one last time as he was introduced. Ty took the mic and said thank you as he walked to the spot where Alonzo had planted himself.

"This is where I will be standing when Josh wins tonight." The crowd cheered and moaned. With nothing to lose, Ty went into his best set of the show. He looked calm, and he made our outfit look good.

Anthony said goodbye to Ty and started to fumble through my introduction. The cameras cut to my parents in the audience, smiling and applauding my opponent.

"You know him, you love him. Here's Josh Blue!"

With a big goofy smile, I tromped onstage wearing the fake glasses with the tape in the middle. Before I took the mic out of the stand, I produced a long, snaking rope from my breast pocket. I spent a minute on improvised magician humor, twirling the rope and ending up with one big knot. Then I went into more callbacks from the show and avoided my written jokes, because whether I won or not, after tonight I was about to hit the road hard. I wanted my fans to hear fresh, new stuff.

Anthony Clark gave me a hug and called Ty back onstage.

"Now, the moment we've all been waiting for, to find out who will be the LAST…COMIC…STANDING…right after this commercial break."

You would think we'd be used to that agony by now, but it hit me in the guts, every time. We waved at our loved ones in the audience, and I asked Anthony if he enjoyed being a dick like this.

Back from the break, Anthony reminded the audience how we had whittled our way down from thousands of comics to Ty and me. "Tonight's winner will receive a talent contract with *NBC* and a one-hour special aired on *Bravo*, but most importantly, the title of LAST COMIC STANDING!"

And then I won.

There was an explosion of confetti and paper streamers. The crowd was on their feet, screaming. You could hear me making a very distinct palsy noise. And then I about vibrated out of my shoes. The happiness message my brain sent my body was almost unbearable, making me lose more of my fine motor skills.

My parents took the stage, followed by all the other contestants from the show. My fine motor skills left entirely, and all I could do was hug people. I found Ty in the spot he said he would be and hugged him, too.

It wasn't until much later in my life that I fully understood that my closing joke about the Palsy Punch had brought me full circle from that gangly seventh grade outsider, standing at the bus stop with his Mr. T. lunchbox to the winner of the world's largest comedy contest.

THE AFTERMATH

The day after winning *Last Comic Standing*, I appeared on *Regis & Kelly*, filmed in New York City. I got on a red-eye flight from LAX, leaving the celebration and wrap party early. I'm always bummed to leave a party, and I thought it was especially unfair that all the runners-up got to stay and celebrate my win. But the real work was just beginning.

People think when you reach a certain level of success, things get easier for you. The truth I now know: That's bullshit. I would have to work harder just to maintain this level of success, let alone to move forward to the next thing. I knew I didn't want to be a flash in the pan, the downfall of so many reality show stars. To be successful in this business required constantly being on the road, heading to the next town where people needed to laugh. And so began the comedy grind for the next eighteen years and counting. My new life on a plane.

After I landed in NYC, it was a rush. A town car picked me up and took me to the hotel for a quick shower. I caught a glimpse of myself in the bathroom mirror; I still had makeup on from the big win the day before. It had smeared and run down my face, making me look old and haggard.

Upon arrival at the *Regis & Kelly* studio, they took me directly to makeup, prepped me a bit for the show, and then I was on. Emeril Lagasse was guest hosting. He was very nice, but I felt a little ripped off, because Regis wasn't there. Kelly was as sweet as you can imagine. She gave me a big hug, and I was amazed such an embrace could come from such a petite person. She's so tiny. When I hugged her, it was like hugging myself; I had to check to make sure she was in there.

Later that year, I was invited back to be on the show. I'd won a Relly Award for Best Reality Show Winner. I eventually shot the award with a pellet gun, like I do with all my trophies.

On the plane headed back to L.A. to guest on *The Ellen DeGeneres Show*, I was in a weird spot. My body was exhausted, but my brain was racing. These big adrenaline bursts mixed with heavy drinking and smoking copious amounts of marijuana were especially hard on the body. All that, followed by the lonely downtime of a six-hour flight. It was surreal and sad to be spending so much time alone.

I was excited to be on *The Ellen DeGeneres Show*. Her writing and timing as a stand-up are impeccable, and she has such a lovable energy. She invited me to be the first stand-up to ever perform on her show. I had a five-minute set, and I mentally went over the jokes I would do, but I was more concerned with not embarrassing myself in front of one of my idols.

I have a tendency to nerd out when I meet a comedian I admire. I will quote my favorite jokes of theirs to them, and I wanted to avoid that with Ellen. She knows how good she is; that's why I was about to appear on *her* TV show.

I slept a few hours on the flight, and upon arrival it was another town car, hotel, and shower; then it was off to the studio. In my dressing room, I found another gift basket. There was a bathrobe and some boxer briefs with the show's logo on them. I thought about putting them on and stumbling around in them, but then I remembered I hadn't performed yet, and she could still change her mind.

I was excited to see who else was on the show. I poked my

head out of the door to see fucking Sting walk by. Put on the red light! He was there to shoot another episode that would air later in the week. I wanted to ask him if I could have his Ellen robe; we're about the same size, but I worried he would tell me not to stand so close to him. Either way, it didn't look like he had a message in a bottle for me.

A security guard came to the door and said the other guest on the show, Sandra Oh, wanted to meet me. I was curious why she would beckon little old me to her dressing room. I tentatively followed the guard to her door like this was some sort of prank.

I knocked softly and opened it. There was the beautiful Sandra Oh, smiling. "I wanted to meet you," she said. "You look a lot like my boyfriend." *Whaaat? You mean I have a chance?*

Someone with a headset came and told me the studio audience was all set and ready. The show started, and Ellen introduced me. I was more excited than nervous. I always try to perform to the audience at hand and not think about the millions of viewers whose laughter I can't hear. I did my five minutes, and the audience loved me. When I was done, I took a bow and walked over to sit with Ellen. I was relieved that I crushed, and now I got to chat with one of my top five comics of all time.

She was all smiles and gave me a big hug. She asked me questions about my artwork and had pictures of some of my paintings. I playfully batted back any questions she threw at me with my crooked little smile. She and the audience ate it up. We went to commercial break, and I had four minutes of alone time with her—microphones off.

"You're so funny. I don't know why I picked you to be the first one to do stand-up on my show, but I'm glad I did. I love your phone number joke." And then she told my joke.

I didn't think it could get any better than it already was, but now Ellen was quoting my material back to me.

Four days after my win, I was finally home, and I could properly celebrate. The city of Denver had organized a parade in my honor. It was like I had won the Super Bowl of jokes, and I kicked off the parade by taking the maiden voyage up the Comedy Works' new elevator—finally making them ADA compliant, alongside then-Mayor Hickenlooper. No one would ever have to carry a wheelchair down the stairs again.

We stood awkwardly in the hot elevator for about ten minutes while the camera crews upstairs got ready for our entrance. Hickenlooper congratulated me on all my triumphs, and after a long moment, said, "Wow Josh Blue, you really smell like kind bud."

I laughed and offered him a hit as the elevator started to move, but he declined. You can see in the pictures, we're still laughing about it as we got off the elevator. The Mayor gave me the key to the city and declared that day in Denver's history as Josh Blue Day.

The parade was short; possibly the shortest in the history of parades, so we went around the block again. I got to ride atop a fire truck, jumping like a booboo monkey, making the firefighters nervous. Scott Johnson drove in a tiny Go Kart, like a circus bear. Comedy Works had printed up masks of my face for people to wear; it was terrifying to see an army of me cheering me on.

After the parade, I dismounted the fire truck in an ocean of hugs and high fives. Riding the euphoria, I made my way to the Go Karts for an ill-advised test drive through the city. As you might assume, I do not have my driver's license, but I stomped on the accelerator and tore out of the parking lot—directly into the path of an oncoming car. They slammed on their brakes and screeched to a stop, inches from my face. I giggled and drove off, away from the gasps of fans who almost witnessed me die on Josh Blue Day.

I've been doing over two hundred shows a year since I won *Last Comic Standing*, eighteen years ago. Many things have changed, including me. I continued touring the world playing soccer until Coach Hoffman retired me in 2015. I continue to make art and have had nine gallery shows and sold over one hundred pieces. I've been married and divorced, and came out of that storm with the two most amazing accomplishments of my life: my son Simon and my daughter Seika, not to mention my amazing partner Mercy.

People still ask me if *Last Comic Standing* was the biggest success of my life. It is not.

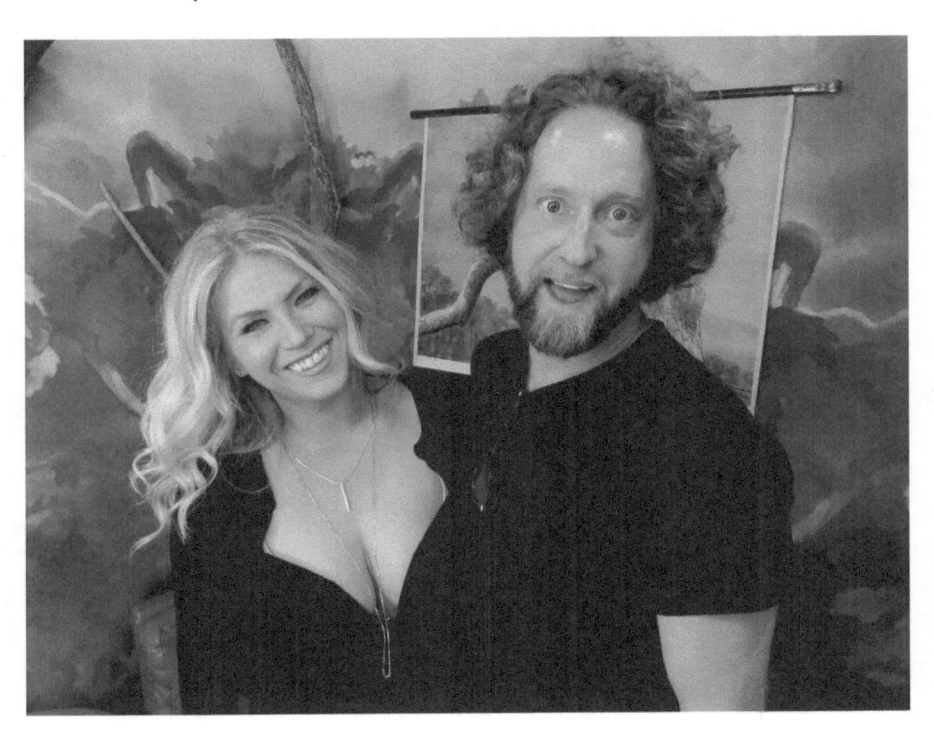

290 | *Something To Stare At*

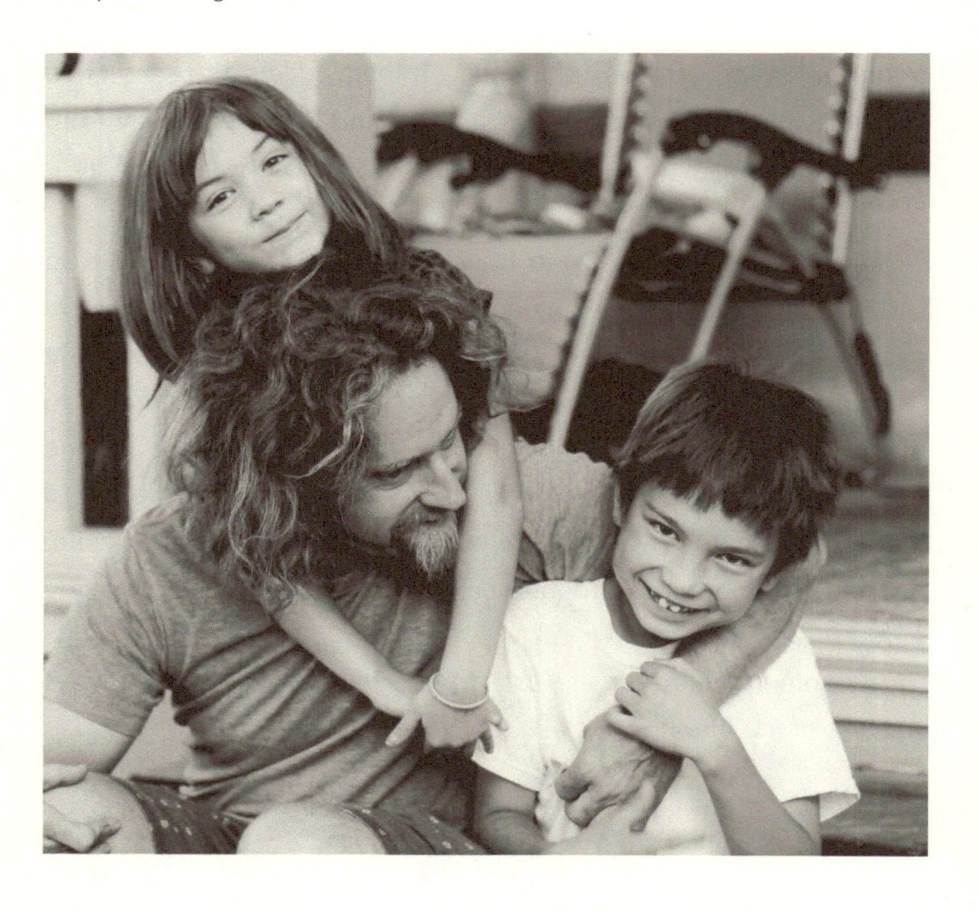

ABOUT THE AUTHOR

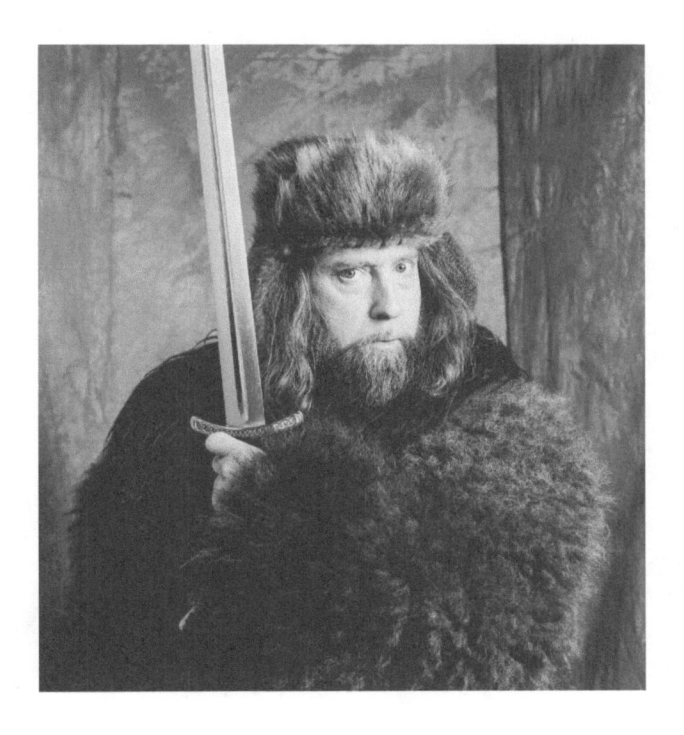

Following his groundbreaking win on *NBC's Last Comic Standing* in 2006, Josh Blue has become one of America's top touring comedians and performs over 200 shows a year, spreading laughter and smashing stereotypes of people with disabilities. Josh represented the U.S. as a member of the Paralympic soccer team. An accomplished painter and sculptor, he holds solo and group exhibitions. Josh lives in Denver, Colorado, with his patient partner Mercy, his clever kids Simon and Seika, and even more clever cats, Remy and Arlo.

JOSHBLUE.COM

Made in United States
Troutdale, OR
08/09/2025